# The Heart of Justice

# The Heart of Justice

## Care Ethics and Political Theory

Daniel Engster

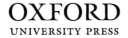
OXFORD
UNIVERSITY PRESS

# OXFORD

UNIVERSITY PRESS

Great Clarendon Street, Oxford OX2 6DP

Oxford University Press is a department of the University of Oxford.
It furthers the University's objective of excellence in research, scholarship,
and education by publishing worldwide in

Oxford  New York

Auckland   Cape Town  Dar es Salaam   Hong Kong   Karachi
Kuala Lumpur  Madrid  Melbourne  Mexico City   Nairobi
New Delhi  Shanghai  Taipei  Toronto
With offices in
Argentina  Austria  Brazil  Chile  Czech Republic  France  Greece
Guatemala  Hungary  Italy  Japan  South Korea  Poland  Portugal
Singapore  Switzerland  Thailand  Turkey  Ukraine  Vietnam

Oxford is a registered trade mark of Oxford University Press
in the UK and in certain other countries

Published in the United States
by Oxford University Press Inc., New York

© Daniel Engster 2007

The moral rights of the author have been asserted

Database right Oxford University Press (maker)

Reprinted 2009

ISBN 978-0-19-956249-7

Printed in the United Kingdom by
Lightning Source UK Ltd., Milton Keynes

To my parents, David and Helen Engster, and Julia Landois

# Acknowledgments

Care theory offers an important new perspective on morality and politics. From the early works of Carol Gilligan and Nel Noddings to the more recent contributions of Joan Tronto, Eva Kittay, Virginia Held, and others, care theorists have challenged existing assumptions about the nature of morality and politics and offered fresh insights into these fields of study. While I have long admired the ideas of care theorists, I nonetheless have found it difficult when teaching courses on contemporary political theories to find any single book on care theory that could stand alongside works such as John Rawls's *A Theory of Justice* or Robert Nozick's *Anarchy, State, and Utopia* as a general statement of the nature and aims of a caring government. Joan Tronto's *Moral Boundaries* (1993) persuasively demonstrates that care theory can be applied to political theory, but she devotes only the last chapter to a brief discussion of the institutions and policies of a caring society. The recent works of Eva Kittay (1999), Nel Noddings (2002), and Virginia Held (2006) further outline some of the policies of a caring government, but their arguments, too, offer something less than a full account of the basic institutions and policies of a caring society. As I began to work on care theory, I also discovered that many professional political theorists know little, if anything, about care theory. Most have at least heard of Gilligan's *In A Different Voice*, but beyond this work, few have much knowledge of the field of care theory.

For these reasons, I decided to write a book on care ethics and political theory that might help to introduce the ideas of care theorists to a broader audience and spell out more concretely the institutions and policies of a caring society. With this goal in mind, I chose to reformulate care theory in terms of an analytical theory of justice. I begin with a definition of caring, outline a theory of moral obligation that shows why we should care for others, and then draw out the logical implications of these ideas for domestic politics, economics, international relations, and culture. While care theorists have sometimes been wary of traditional justice frameworks, I argue that care theorists' usual objections to justice frameworks are not very strong (see Introduction). Moreover, I consider it important to reframe care ethics in terms of a theory of justice in order to make it more accessible to readers outside the field and more applicable to practical politics.

In translating care ethics into a theory of justice, I remove it somewhat from the feminist context in which it has developed. I nonetheless owe a great debt to the feminist care theorists who have established this field of moral and political thought. This book simply would not have been possible without the works of Carol Gilligan, Nel Noddings, Sara Ruddick, Joan Tronto, Virginia Held, Eva Kittay, Marilyn Friedman, Julie White, and many other care theorists. Studying the works of these care theorists not only changed the way I think about politics, but also the way I think about myself and my relations to others.

I am grateful to the many people who have read and provided me helpful comments on various chapters of this book. I especially want to thank Katy Arnold, Doug Dow, Nancy Folbre, Kathleen Hancock, Jim Lasko, Traci Levy, Hilde Lindemann, Joan Tronto, Jorge Valadez, and the anonymous reviewers of this book. Numerous conference discussants and panelists also provided useful feedback on early versions of my chapters. Joshua Doyen provided me with some much needed research support in the final stages of preparing my manuscript. I would also like to thank Dominic Byatt at Oxford University Press for showing faith and perseverance in finding readers for my manuscript and bringing my book to press, Lizzy Suffling and Kate Hind for their editorial work, and Richard Preston for proofreading my book.

My greatest debt is to Julia Landois, whom I lived with and loved during the gestation and writing of this book. Hardly a day went by that I did not discuss some of my arguments with her, and her feedback was always invaluable. More generally, she supported me during the difficult times that accompanied my writing of this book and showed unflagging faith in me and my project. She is in every thought in this book, and contributed many of them.

I would like to thank the University of Texas at San Antonio for providing me with a semester research leave to work on this book. My department chairs, Richard Gambitta and Mansour El-Kikhia, and colleagues were also generous in their support of my research.

I would also like to thank the National Endowment of the Humanities for providing me with a Faculty Research Award that allowed me to take a semester off from my teaching and service obligations to work on this book. Any views, findings, conclusions, or recommendations expressed in this publication do not necessarily reflect those of the National Endowment for the Humanities.

I would finally like to thank the following publishers for permission to use revised versions or portions of my earlier articles. An earlier version of Chapter One appeared as 'Rethinking Care Theory: The Practice of Caring and the Obligation to Care', *Hypatia*, 20(3) (Summer 2005), pp. 50–74, published by Indiana University Press. An early attempt to outline a political theory of caring appeared as 'Care Ethics and Natural Law Theory: Toward an Institutional Political Theory of Caring', *The Journal of Politics*, 66(1) (February 2004), pp. 113–35, published by Blackwell Publishing.

# Contents

# Introduction

Caring is at the heart of human existence. Infants and small children would not survive or develop their basic capabilities without the care of parents or some sort of parenting figures. Few adults would live out the full extent of their natural lives without the care of family, friends, and others. We all depend upon the care of others during sickness, disability, and frail old age, and most of us rely on family and friends to help us meet our needs and function even during times of relative health and vigor. Caring further sustains society and makes civil life possible. If no one cared for the young, society would cease to exist within a couple of generations. If no one cared for the sick, old, and disabled, our social bonds would begin to fray. In a world without care, human life would be truly 'poor, solitary, nasty, brutish, and short'—if it existed at all.

Despite the importance of caring to human life and society, Western philosophers have generally paid little attention to it in developing their moral and political philosophies.[1] Moral and political theories have been developed around conceptions of the good life, divine law, natural rights, autonomy, and utility, but caring has usually been treated as a sub-moral and pre-political activity (Tronto 1996: 139–42). Aristotle briefly discusses caring within the home at the beginning of his *Politics*, but then proceeds to argue that the main substance of morality and politics exists outside and beyond these activities (Aristotle 1995: 8–10, 1252a–1253a). St Thomas Aquinas acknowledges the importance of caring in sustaining and reproducing human life, but orients his political philosophy around religious ends. Modern liberal theorists from John Locke to John Rawls have generally focused their accounts of justice on protecting and promoting individual autonomy and equality while for the most part relegating caring to the private sphere.

[1] Scottish Enlightenment thinkers, such as Francis Hutcheson, David Hume, and Adam Smith, outlined moral and political philosophies that share some similarities with the ideas of care theorists (see Baier 1994: 51–94; Tronto 1993: 25–59). Mary Wollstonecraft, too, incorporated caring into her political thought (Engster 2001).

1

This book challenges these long-standing assumptions about care and justice by placing caring at the center of a moral and political theory. Because human beings universally depend upon one another for care, we all have moral obligations to care for others in need. While we can fulfill some of our obligations to others through personal caring relationships, we can fulfill many others only through collective caring institutions and policies. Our moral obligations to care for others thus generate collective responsibilities to organize our political, economic, international, and cultural institutions at least in part to support caring practices and care for individuals in need.

My argument builds upon the work of a group of mostly feminist thinkers who over the past twenty-five years or so have developed moral and political theories based upon caring. Carol Gilligan (1982) and Nel Noddings (1984) laid the foundations for care ethics, arguing that caring represents a unique mode of relating to others and solving moral problems that has generally been ignored by Western philosophers. Rather than approaching moral questions in terms of rights, utility or other ideals, Gilligan and Noddings argued that care ethics aims to meet the concrete needs of individuals in context-specific and responsive ways. In recent years, numerous other theorists have built upon, amended, and expanded these ideas in order to elaborate more clearly what it means to care for others and to explain how caring might be integrated into public policy.[2]

Care theory as a general body of thought nonetheless has a number of gaps and ambiguities that have limited its development as a moral and political theory. Critics have argued, for example, that the concept of caring is too vague to provide adequate grounding to moral and political theory. Early care theorists defined caring primarily as a manner of relating to others through sympathy, attentiveness, and responsiveness. Owen Flanagan and Jonathan Adler note, however, that it is not enough for care theorists simply to say that people should sympathize with others or attend to their particular needs and circumstances: 'We have been told nothing about [care ethics] until we are told what features of situations context-sensitive people pick out as morally salient, what

---

[2] In addition to the early works of Gilligan (1982) and Noddings (1984), some of the most important works in the field include Baier (1994, 1997), Blustein (1991), Bowden (1997), Bubeck (1995), Clement (1996), Darwall (2002), Diller (1996), Fineman (2004), Folbre (2001), Friedman (1993), Grimshaw (1986), Groenhout (2004), Harrington (2000), Held (1993, 2006), Kittay (1999), Kittay and Feder (2002), Noddings (1992, 2002), Robinson (1999), Ruddick (1989), Schwarzenbach (1987, 1996), Sevenhuijsen (1998), Slote (2001), Tronto (1993), Walker (1998), West (1997), White (2000), and White and Tronto (2004).

weightings they put on these different features, and so on.... We simply need to know more, in a detailed way... about exactly what it is they care about' (Flanagan and Adler 1983: 592). While recent care theorists have sharpened their definitions of caring, Flanagan and Adler's core criticism still applies (see Chapter 1). Caring is often defined in ways that leaves ambiguous what we do when we care for others.

Care theorists have also outlined only partial accounts of why we should care for others.[3] Some care theorists suggest that theories of obligation for caring are beside the point since caring arises naturally from an innate sense of sympathy or compassion or at least represents a fundamental ground of morality beyond which there can be no further justification (Donovan 1996; Luke 1996; Noddings 1984; Warren 2000: 111–13). While I agree that the sentiments of sympathy and compassion are important in motivating caring behaviors (and even devote an entire chapter—Chapter 5—to discussing how these sentiments can be culti-vated), I nonetheless consider a rational theory of obligation for caring to be important for a number of reasons.[4] First, even if the disposition to care is innate, it still needs to be nurtured through appropriate childrearing practices, education, and other forms of socialization. Under unsuitable conditions, children may not develop the capacity for sympathy or com-passion at all. If the sentiments of sympathy and compassion must be actively cultivated, in turn, then some reason must be given for why we should cultivate them. It might be argued, after all, that aggression and prejudice are also natural sentiments, but care theorists certainly do not recommend that we attempt to develop and strengthen them. Why, then, cultivate sympathy and compassion but not aggression and prejudice? A theory of obligation provides an answer to this question. We should cultivate the former sentiments but not the latter because the former are consistent with what we can rationally show to be our moral obligations while the latter are not.

A rational theory of obligation is important in other ways as well. Even if individuals possess a natural capacity for sympathy and compassion, they may apply these sentiments in highly constricted ways. Racists, nationalists, and others may all behave quite sympathetically toward members of their group but reprehensibly toward others. A caring theory of obligation explains why we should expand our sympathies beyond our immediate circle of family and friends to encompass all human beings

---

[3] The most important work on this topic has been done by Fineman (2004), Friedman (1993), and Kittay (1999). Their theories are discussed in Chapter 1.

[4] I develop this argument in more detail in Chapter 1.

in need. Tom Regan pointedly asks: 'What are the resources within the ethic of care that can move people to consider the ethics of their dealings with individuals who stand outside the *existing circle* of their valued interpersonal relationships?' (Regan 1991: 95). An answer to this question is important in developing a moral and political theory of caring, since care theory might otherwise seem to justify nothing more than a narrow familial or group morality (Barry 1995: 252–5).

A third gap in the literature on care ethics relates to the institutions and policies that follow from our obligation to care for others. In recent years, care theorists have identified a number of social and political policies associated with caring but have for the most part discussed and defended these policies in a piecemeal fashion (Fineman 2004; Folbre 2001; Harrington 2000; Kittay 1999; Noddings 2002; Robinson 1999; Tronto 1993). No general account of the basic institutions and policies of a caring society has yet been proposed.[5] Care theorists have also thus far failed to address adequately the challenge of multiculturalism. Since most societies today are populated by individuals with diverse cultural and religious views, it is important to situate care ethics in relation to these diverse worldviews if it is to have broad relevance and appeal as a general moral and political theory.

This book develops a moral and political theory of caring that addresses these shortcomings. In comparison with existing works on care theory, it makes four distinctive contributions. (a) It outlines and defends a definition of caring that can more satisfactorily guide the development of a moral and political theory. (b) It develops a theory of obligation for caring that explains why we ought to care for others. (c) It extends existing accounts of care theory to identify the basic institutions and policies of a caring society across the domains of politics, economics, international relations, and culture. (d) It places care ethics in dialogue with diverse cultural and religious traditions and uses it to address the challenges of multicultural justice, cultural relativism, and international human rights.

Altogether, this book outlines a theory of justice based upon the practice of caring. The main goal is to bring the insights of care theory more directly to bear on contemporary moral and political debates about the nature of a just society. Since John Rawls published *A Theory of Justice*

normative

---

[5] Rawls organizes his theory of justice around the basic institutions or basic structure of society, by which he means 'the political constitution and the principal economic and social arrangements' (Rawls 1999b: 6). I follow suit in describing the principal political, economic, and cultural arrangements of a caring society. The limitation of this approach is that I do not discuss many particular social policies and issues, such as care theory's approach to abortion, animal rights, or crime and punishment.

(1971), political theorists have outlined numerous accounts of a just society, representing libertarian, communitarian, market socialist, natural law, and other perspectives. This book situates care theory alongside these other theories as an alternative vision of a just society.

More fundamentally, the book argues that the principles of care theory are central to *any* adequate theory of justice. There would be no indi- vidual liberty or equality, community values or good life without the caring practices necessary to sustain and foster human life and society. As such, the aims and virtues of caring may be said to precede and underlie all other theories of justice. No theory of justice can be said to be consistent or complete without integrating the institutional and policy commitments of care theory. Care theory nonetheless does not completely subsume all other theories of justice. My account of care theory describes a minimal and incomplete theory of justice that does not provide guidance on many policy questions or make specific rec- ommendations about the nature of the good life. Other theories of jus- tice including liberalism, libertarianism, communitarianism, and natural law theory—or other religious or cultural values—might be tacked on to care theory to address issues such as the proper role of religion in public life or the appropriate scope of free speech. Care theory defines only a minimal set of moral and political principles that apply to all people and societies regardless of how else they might choose to organ- ize their private or public lives. In short, while other political theories focus on the ends or goals of society, care theory defines the heart of justice.

*[handwritten margin note: caring comes first]*

## 0.1. Caring and Justice

Since care ethics has traditionally been contrasted with justice theories, my project of developing care ethics into a theory of justice might seem paradoxical. Carol Gilligan, for example, originally developed care ethics in explicit opposition to traditional justice thinking. She defined care ethics as a relational and circumstantial morality that sets aside the justice tradition's usual emphasis on general rules and principles for a more par- ticular and person-based orientation to moral issues (Gilligan 1982: 164– 5). In *Caring: A Feminine Approach to Ethics and Moral Education* (1984), Nel Noddings even more strongly drew out this distinction between caring and justice.[6] She defined caring as engrossment in the particular wants

---

[6] Noddings has revised her position in more recent writings, now arguing that social and political institutions can manifest and support caring in important ways (2002: 22–4).

and desires of others and justice as a commitment to abstract principles and rules (1984: 24, 36). Because caring entails personal engrossment in particular persons, she argued it could never be faithfully represented through a general theory of justice or manifested in political institutions (18, 103).

While the distinction between care and justice is perhaps one of the best-known features of care ethics, numerous theorists have argued that it does not stand up to critical scrutiny (Bubeck 1995: 189–241; Flanagan and Adler 1983; Grimshaw 1986: 205–11; Kymlicka 1990: 276–84; Okin 1989b). Susan Okin and Diemut Bubeck argue, for instance, that both Gilligan and Noddings make use of some implicit and unacknowledged moral principles in outlining their accounts of care ethics that can be formulated into a justice theory (Bubeck 1995: 189–241; Okin 1990). Jean Grimshaw and others have likewise noted that general principles and rules need not be objectifying or impersonal in the way that Gilligan and Noddings portray them, but instead can serve as general guidelines or considerations 'to take into account when deciding what is the right thing to do' in particular situations (1986: 208; Bubeck 1995: 208–14). Some guidelines or principles would further seem necessary for defining the nature of caring and distinguishing good forms of care from bad. If caring is defined as a wholly contextual moral orientation, it may be difficult to differentiate it from paternalistic, exploitative, and other relations that may masquerade as caring (Friedman 1993: 126–31; Goodin 1996). An overly intrusive, controlling, or even abusive parent or partner might justify his or her behavior in terms of his or her caring concern for his or her loved ones.

Care theorists have similarly argued that Gilligan's and Noddings's personal and apolitical approach to caring can lead to some uncaring conclusions. Most basically, personal approaches to caring fail to take into account the web of social relationships in which any particular caring relationship necessarily exists (Kittay 1999). Since individuals can usually only care effectively for others if provided some sort of support or accommodation by others, theories that focus narrowly on personal caring relations fail to recognize the important role that social institutions and policies can play in fostering good caring relations. Claudia Card further notes that strictly personal approaches to caring render 'as ethically insignificant our relationships with most people in the world, because we do not know them and never will', and Joan Tronto adds that too much emphasis on personal caring 'could quickly become a way to argue that everyone should cultivate one's own garden, and let others take care of themselves' (Card 1990: 102; Tronto 1993: 103, 171). Virginia Held likewise argues that valorizing personal caring without attending to larger issues of social justice can serve to justify existing care arrangements that place the burden of care work primarily on women and minority groups without providing them with adequate recognition or compensation (Held 2006: 16). As even Noddings now acknowledges, care theory needs to be connected to a theory of justice and applied to social institutions if it is to avoid these shortcomings (Noddings 2002: 22–4).

*communities*

## 0.2. Caring and Other Contemporary Justice Theories

Care theory may not be distinct from other justice theories in form, but it is distinct in substance (Bubeck 1995: 187). While some other justice theories partially recognize and support some caring practices, only care theory organizes morality and politics around the goal of supporting caring practices and ensuring adequate care for all individuals. Since one of the main aims of this book is to demonstrate the distinctive nature of care theory, it may be useful here at the outset to compare care theory in general terms with other justice theories. The remainder of the book develops the institutional and policy commitments of care theory in detail, but this discussion can at least serve as a general road map for situating care theory in the landscape of contemporary political theory.

In contemporary Western political theory, liberal theories represent the most influential accounts of justice. The most basic difference between liberalism and care theory lies in their different premises (Clement 1996: 11–20; Friedman 1993: 221–30; Hirschmann 1996: 157–80; Noddings 2002: 69–117). Liberal theories of justice generally assume the equality and autonomy of individual human beings. In their classical form, these theories begin by imagining a number of equal and autonomous individuals coming together to form a political society usually through a hypothetical social contract. In liberal frameworks, principles of justice are generally determined by imagining what all individuals would reasonably agree to endorse in the original contract, and obligations are said to arise strictly from individuals' free and voluntary consent. Care theory, by contrast, begins with individuals already existing in society and dependent upon one another for their survival, development, and social functioning, and highlights the unchosen obligations we all have toward others by virtue of our interdependency. Because we are all born into a state of dependency and depend upon others more or less throughout our lives, all capable individuals have obligations to care for others in need regardless of our explicit or tacit consent.

These different premises of liberalism and care theory give rise to important differences in these theories' orientations toward justice. Most liberal theories are concerned primarily with protecting the equal liberty and rights of individuals. Many liberal theorists argue that the commitment to equal liberty and rights includes some forms of support for people in need, but they have usually conceived of this support in terms of unemployment.insurance, disability subsidies, and other policies related to market failures. Few liberal theorists have made support for personal caregiving an integral part of their theories. In *A Theory of Justice*, for example, John Rawls says nothing about parenting leaves or public child-care even though he acknowledges the importance of healthy families and good childcare for the maintenance and reproduction of a just society (Okin 1989a: 89–109, 1994). Family and personal care activities remain for him, as for most liberals, a private responsibility outside the proper scope of a theory of justice (Kittay 1999: 76). Care theory, by contrast, makes public support for parenting, education, health care, elder care, and the like the main substance of justice. While care theory also supports some individual liberties—specifically those rights and liberties that are necessary to ensure that all individuals are able to give and receive adequate care—it does not endorse all the rights and liberties usually endorsed by liberal thinkers.

Despite these differences between care theory and liberalism, Susan Okin suggests that the commitments of care theory are already encompassed within the philosophical framework of liberalism and need only to be drawn out by reworking liberal premises (1989b). She demonstrates her claim by reinterpreting Rawls's theory of justice to highlight the caring elements within it. Rawls premises his account of justice upon an imaginative construct called the 'original position'. In the original position, individuals are deprived of all knowledge about their race, class, sex, tastes, and abilities, and asked to identify general principles of justice that they can all reasonably agree to follow once they enter into society and discern their particular attributes. Rawls explains that the basic idea of the original position is to provide a starting place for thinking about justice that reflects 'men's desire to treat one another not as means only but as ends in themselves' (Rawls 1999b: 156). Okin argues that Rawls's theory, properly understood, contains a commitment 'to *caring* about each and every other as much as about ourselves' (1989b: 245–6). Because individuals in the original position cannot know what characteristics they will have in society, they are forced to think about the interests of all other individuals and endorse justice principles that treat all others fairly

While I agree with Okin that liberalism is compatible with care theory, and that a liberal account of justice can be tacked on to a caring theory of government, her suggestion that all the commitments of care theory can be derived from strictly liberal premises seems dubious. Even if Rawls's theory can justify a form of caring among *some* individuals, it does not support caring for *all* individuals (Kittay 1999: 75–113). Rawls, like other liberal theorists, premises his account of justice on an agreement among equal and autonomous individuals—situated in this case in the original position. In outlining the premises of the original position, Rawls even stipulates that individuals should be assumed to have physical and psychological capabilities within the 'normal range', setting aside for 'later' the question of how to address the special needs of dependent individuals and their caregivers (Kittay 1999: 80, 88; Rawls 1996: 272 n. 10; 1999b: 83–4). Excluded from the original position are thus all those individuals who have special survival and developmental needs such as children, the frail elderly, disabled persons, and sick individuals, and the special needs of those individuals who care for these dependent individuals. Kittay writes in this regard, 'While the Rawlsian construct allows for the possibility that a representative *may* imagine himself or herself as a dependent or having responsibility for a dependent's care, it does not necessitate that a representative *will* do so when choosing the principles of a well-ordered society. Dependents do not form an obvious constituency within the Rawlsian construct' (Kittay 1999: 86).[7] Kittay's critique is, however, too weak. If the purpose of the Rawlsian contract is to achieve a fair agreement among the representatives in the original position, and these representatives are (in accordance with liberal premises) all assumed to be autonomous and equal individuals, then it would seem illicit for these individuals to raise concerns about caregiving and dependency. These concerns are by definition outside the scope of the original position and liberal justice, representing the particular concerns of particular individuals. One could, of course, radically change the assumptions of Rawls's original position in order to include caring and dependency within it, but then one would be changing the liberal premises upon which Rawls's theory rests. The

---

[7] In *A Theory of Justice*, Rawls does argue that the individuals in the original position should be considered heads of households. But Kittay notes: 'Although Rawls speaks of each person in the OP [original position] caring about the welfare of some in the next [generation], the concern is with a scarcity of resources across generations, not the care of dependents.... Rawls does not introduce representation by heads of households to solve problems arising from dependency, and in *Political Liberalism* Rawls abandons the idea altogether' (1999: 85).

original position would model not so much what it means for individuals to treat one another as autonomous and equal individuals as what it means for individuals to recognize their inescapable interdependency on one another. Where individual autonomy and equality is the starting place for a theory of justice, it is at least difficult to see how full recognition for caring and dependency can be included as basic matters of justice (Fraser and Gordon 2002; Kittay 1999: 110–13; Young 2002).

Care theory shares more in common with communitarian political philosophies. Both care theory and communitarian theories emphasize the interconnectedness of human beings and the nonvoluntary nature of many of our moral obligations (Etzioni 1993; MacIntyre 1981; Sandel 1982; Taylor 1985). Many (but certainly not all) communitarian theorists further support some caring public policies such as subsidies for parenting leaves and childcare. Care theory nonetheless also departs from communitarian theories in important ways (Friedman 1993: 231–55; Kittay 2001). Many communitarian thinkers recognize no independent moral criteria for judging the legitimacy of social institutions and traditions outside the community.[8] The institutions and traditions of the community define the 'rightful expectations and obligations' placed upon their members (MacIntyre 1981: 204–5). One might draw upon the values and traditions of one's community to challenge certain practices or institutions, but there is no outside 'moral starting point' for critical reflection (MacIntyre 1981: 205). Care theory, by contrast, identifies the practice of caring as an independent moral criterion for judging the validity of institutions and traditions. It supports existing communal institutions and practices that facilitate decent caring relations, but challenges or suggests reforms to existing institutions and practices that hinder them (Kittay 2001).

Care theory also has different aims from communitarian theories. Communitarian theorists are generally concerned with strengthening communal ties and promoting social solidarity as ends in themselves. Care theory aims more basically at ensuring a basic threshold of adequate care for all individuals. It is not so much concerned with promoting community or social solidarity as making sure that children, sick persons, disabled individuals, the elderly, and others in need receive the care they need to survive and function in society. In pursuing these goals, care theory does

---

[8] The 'new communitarians', including Amitai Etzioni, Benjamin Barber, and others, combine their communitarian views with a universal account of human nature and a commitment to individual rights (The Responsive Communitarian Platform 1998). Richard Rorty goes perhaps the furthest in developing a communitarian philosophy that is explicitly and unapologetically ethnocentric (Rorty 1989).

support a number of communal institutions including families, schools, and community centers, but the goal is to ensure adequate care for all individuals rather than to strengthen community per se. Perhaps most importantly, care theory opposes any measures that might strengthen community at the cost of adequate care for all individuals.

Among contemporary political theories, my account of care theory bears the closest resemblance to certain variants of natural law theory. Consistent with the natural law tradition, I suggest that the basic principles of morality can be identified by reflecting upon the nature of human existence and the practices necessary to sustain human life as we know it. Since we all depend upon the care of others to survive and achieve basic social functioning, we all should reasonably be able to recognize a duty to care for others in need. Governments can help us to fulfill our moral duties by creating an institutional framework for supporting and accommodating caring practices and caring for those in need. As such, governments function in care theory much as they do in natural law theory to facilitate moral relations among people, sustain human life and society, and promote a common good.

The main difference between my account of care theory and other natural law theories stems from the more minimal nature of the common good, or level of flourishing, supported by care theory. Classical natural law theorists such as Aristotle and St Thomas Aquinas argued that there exists a single best life for human beings, defined as a life of philosophical or religious contemplation, that governments should promote among their citizens. Contemporary natural law thinkers such as Martha Nussbaum and John Finnis have argued more modestly that governments should aim only to provide all individuals with the opportunity to develop a broad array of capabilities or basic values associated with the good life, including artistic appreciation, play, knowledge, political participation, and religious worship (Finnis 1980; Nussbaum 2000).[9] My account of care theory suggests more modestly still that governments should function primarily to provide all individuals the opportunity to satisfy their basic needs, develop and sustain their innate capabilities for sensation, mobility, emotion, imagination, reason, language, and sociability, and live as much as possible free from unwanted suffering and pain. These more minimal goals avoid Nussbaum's and Finnis's contentious claims about what makes human life worthwhile (art, play, political participation, and religion) and focus more fundamentally on the basic

---

[9] Nussbaum's theory is further discussed in Chapter 1.

goals (survival, development, and basic social functioning) that make human life possible.

Care theory can thus ultimately be best characterized as a minimal capability theory or needs-based philosophy.[10] Consistent with the capability approach, the goal of care theory is to help individuals achieve a basic level of social functioning. In this regard, it recognizes that different individuals may have different levels of needs and that different bundles of goods and services may suffice for helping different individuals to achieve adequate levels of functioning in different circumstances. It further aims to involve individuals in identifying and interpreting their needs whenever possible, thus avoiding the danger of paternalism or commodifying needs (Tronto 1993: 137–41; White 2000). More in line with needs-based philosophies, however, care theory defines the level of functioning in a fairly minimal way. It does not take a position on what constitutes a 'truly human' life—as Nussbaum does—but rather supports the caring practices that are necessary for enabling individuals to survive, develop, and achieve basic functioning in society (Nussbaum 2000: 72). Care theory finally departs from both the capabilities approach and needs-based philosophies in its normative grounding. The duty to care for others derives not from human needs in themselves or any philosophical claims about the inherent dignity or worth of all human beings but instead from our inevitable dependency on others and the web of caring relationships that sustains us.

## 0.3. Caring, Gender, and Feminism

Care theory has been developed primarily by feminist philosophers and addresses a number of concerns that are especially relevant to women. As such, it may be said to represent a feminist approach of justice. It is important to be clear, however, about what exactly this means. Carol Gilligan originally portrayed care ethics as a moral perspective closely associated with women's moral voice. Although she noted that the care perspective is not unique to women, she claimed to find an empirical correlation between care ethics and the mode of moral thinking most often used by

[10] On the capabilities approach, see the works of Amartya Sen and Martha Nussbaum, especially Sen (1999) and Nussbaum (2001). Two more recent and important needs-based philosophies are Braybrooke (1987) and Wiggins (1998). A good discussion of the basic needs and capabilities approaches can be found in Reader (2006).

women (Gilligan 1982: 2; 1986: 327). Subsequent psychological research, however, has found this correlation to be fairly weak (Jaffee and Hyde 2000).[11] Women are on average only slightly more likely than men to use care thinking rather than a justice framework in addressing moral issues. While care theory may be a *feminist* morality, therefore, it does not appear to represent a distinctively *feminine* morality.

Many feminist theorists have further been wary of valorizing the connection between women and caring. If caring is portrayed as a distinctively feminine orientation or practice, then care theory might seem to endorse the traditional division of care work along gender lines (O'Neill 1992; Puka 1990, 1991). It might be suggested that women should perform the majority of care work in society because they are naturally inclined toward these activities. Virginia Held argues in this regard that feminist defenders of an ethic of care should make clear 'why men as well as women should value caring relations and should share equally in cultivating them' (Held 2006: 22). My argument overlaps with feminist theory on this point. In Chapter 1, I depict caring as a generic practice that is equally accessible to both men and women and universally obligatory for all capable human beings. In Chapters 2, 3, and 4, I argue that caring should be placed at the center of a public conception of justice and applied to the basic institutions and policies of society so that more support and accommodation is provided for care work. In Chapter 5, I describe a number of cultural reforms that governments might enact in the areas of family life, education, and the media in order to encourage both men and women—but especially men—to be more open to caring. In general, then, my theory supports a more egalitarian distribution of care work between men and women, more public recognition and support for care work, and a revaluation of caring as a basic human, as opposed to distinctively feminine, activity.

My account of care theory nonetheless departs from most feminist theories in one crucial way. If feminism is defined, as it often is, as a commitment to women's equality and rights, then my account of care theory represents something less than a full feminist theory of justice. Care theory supports the adequate care of all individuals, but not

---

[11] In Chapter 5, I argue that there are nonetheless some reasons for thinking that women may be more positively disposed toward caring than men arising from women's traditional role as the primary caregivers of children. As distinct from Gilligan, however, I do not regard caring as a unique mode of moral reasoning involving situational and relational thinking but rather suggest that women may be more caring than men in the sense that they are on average more open to sympathizing with others and engaging in caring practices.

necessarily a fully free and egalitarian society (at least in the liberal sense of the term). This is not to deny the importance of women's equality and feminist ideals, but merely to recognize the limits of care theory in supporting them. As Diemut Bubeck argues, if care theory is to remain a cogent perspective, it cannot be treated as a repository for all feminist or other social justice concerns (Bubeck 1995: 250). Its theoretical limits have to be acknowledged. Feminists, liberals, and others who support full equality for women might supplement care theory by drawing on values outside of it that support autonomy and equality for all individuals, but care theory itself does not possess the theoretical resources to support this goal. Care theory nevertheless does go a long way toward supporting more social equality for women, since women's inequality is closely tied to their traditional role as caregivers and the low valuation that caring practices have been accorded by most theories of justice and most societies. As such, care theory (as I develop it) may at least be identified as a *minimal* feminist theory.

## 0.4. The Contemporary Relevance of Care Theory

Even if care theory represents a new approach to justice, one might wonder why there is a need for it. Theories of justice abound in the academic literature, so why care about care theory? The most basic reason to care about care theory is that it describes a basic morality that we are all obligated to follow by virtue of our dependency on others, but that other justice theories have generally neglected. Because we all claim care from others at one time or another during our lives, we owe care to others when we can provide it to them. In addition, there are also a couple of practical political reasons to care about care theory. Care theory can address a number of pressing contemporary social issues that other justice theories are largely ill-equipped to handle.

Most basically, care theory reformulates our ideas about politics to better reflect the new material conditions of contemporary industrial societies. Changes in the nature of work, the influx of more women into the workplace, the increase in single parenthood, the growing elderly population, and other recent demographic and economic developments have rendered traditional approaches to caring in large part inadequate. In many cases, people can no longer engage in the productive work necessary to support themselves and their dependents and at the same time actually provide adequate personal care to themselves and their dependents (Kittay 1999: 129). As a result, many societies now face a crisis of care that leaves many individuals without the nurturance and support they need to survive, develop, and function adequately in society. The personal and social consequences of this care crisis are potentially dire. Individuals who do not receive adequate care are more likely to engage in violence and crime, have difficulty finding and maintaining productive work, suffer depression and anxiety, and experience a number of other personal and health problems.[12] Care theory provides a framework for thinking about and addressing the exigencies of this new social reality. Recognizing that most people need help in order to care adequately for others, care theory assigns government a central role in supporting and accommodating personal caring activities so that all individuals can survive, develop, and function in society at least at adequate levels.

Many governments do, of course, already support some caring policies. I do not mean to suggest that public support for caring is a wholly new idea or that governments currently provide no support for caring activities. Over the past fifty years or so, many European countries, and especially Sweden and the other Scandinavian countries, have enacted many of the caring policies outlined in this book. In doing so, they have pioneered a new form of welfare state that departs in important ways from traditional welfare state ideals. Rather than just protecting their citizens from the uncertainties and failings of the market, they have also extended welfare policies to encompass support and accommodation for various caring activities including childcare, health care, elder care, and the like. The philosophical justification for this new form of caring welfare state nonetheless remains largely underdeveloped (Rothstein 1998). As argued above, liberalism can provide only partial support for many caring policies, and whatever support it does provide can always be challenged from within the liberal tradition on the grounds that it infringes individual freedom. Socialist theories, too, have traditionally been oriented around goals such as establishing worker ownership and control over productive industries rather than ensuring adequate support for caregiving (Folbre 1996; 2001: 209–22). Care theory offers a new theory of justice for this new form of welfare state, justifying a form of

---

[12] The empirical research for this claim is discussed in the body of this work.

government whose central goal is to provide public support for caring activities.

Some of the public policies of countries with caring programs also fail to reflect important caring values. The Swedish government, for instance, has historically used a standardized, one-size-fits-all approach for addressing many of the needs of its citizens (Rothstein 1998: 48, 195–200). Care theory, by contrast, favors a more flexible and decentralized policy approach that offers individuals more choice and input in determining how to care for themselves and others. As such, care theory provides not only a philosophical justification for caring policies but also a framework for examining, critiquing, and extending these policies in order to make them more consistently supportive and accommodating of personal and social caring. Altogether, care theory outlines a theoretical framework for justifying and establishing a new form of welfare state that makes support and accommodation of caring practices its central aim.

Care theory finally supplies a minimal basic morality that can help to mediate the cultural, religious, and moral differences among people. Most societies today are made up of individuals from diverse cultural and religious backgrounds. In our increasingly interdependent and interconnected world, individuals from different religious and cultural traditions are also more and more dependent upon one another to accomplish their goals. Philosophers such as John Rawls, Jurgen Habermas, and Alan Gewirth have proposed moral and political theories to address these challenges, identifying some basic moral principles that they claim people from diverse religious and cultural traditions should all reasonably be able to agree to follow (Gewirth 1978, 1996; Habermas 1984, 1987, 1996; Rawls 1996, 1999*a*, 1999*b*). Care theory similarly identifies a set of common values for intercultural dialogue and cooperation. While different societies and peoples may engage in different sorts of caring practices, there are universal structural features of caring that apply cross-culturally. All individuals have common biological and developmental needs, for example, that must be met in some rather fixed ways if they are to survive, develop, and achieve basic functioning. Since all people depend upon some rather fixed forms of caring for their survival, development, and functioning, all people can be said at least implicitly to recognize caring as a moral good. Care theory should therefore be able to generate a theory of justice that is universally acceptable across different cultural, religious, and moral communities.

## 0.5. Chapter Outline

The arguments outlined above are more fully developed and defended in the following chapters. I begin by outlining a definition of the practice of caring and a theory of obligation for caring, and then describe in some detail the institutions and policies that follow from these premises in the areas of domestic politics, economics, international relations, and culture.

Chapter 1 provides the moral grounding for the rest of the book. I begin by outlining a definition of caring that can guide the development of a general moral and political theory, and then propose a theory of obligation for caring. I argue that we all have obligations to care for others in need because we all have made claims upon others to care for us when in need. The last part of the chapter discusses the rightful distribution of our caring obligations. While we might justifiably show partiality in caring for ourselves and those close to us, I argue that we ultimately have obligations to care for all individuals in need when we can do so.

Chapter 2 applies this account of care theory to the basic political institutions of society. I first address a question that care theorists have not satisfactorily answered: Why should government assume responsibility for supporting caring activities at all? I then outline six principles for establishing and maintaining a caring government, and describe the specific institutions and policies of a caring government. Since any discussion of minimally adequate care will inevitably raise questions about cultural bias, I next discuss the relation between care theory and multiculturalism. I conclude by addressing a number of possible objections to a caring government, including concerns about its costs and moral hazards.

Chapter 3 extends care theory to questions of economic justice. Virginia Held and Nancy Folbre have outlined two important accounts of care and economic justice. While both identify some of the central tenets of a caring economic theory, they focus primarily on supporting and regulating direct care services within the economy. My own approach is broader and more far-reaching, asking how we can best organize our general economic institutions and policies to provide all individuals with a real opportunity to give and receive adequate care. I first take up the question of which economic system (communism, market socialism, market capitalism, etc.) is most conducive to supporting caring practices. I then formulate six general principles for establishing and maintaining a caring economic system, and describe in some detail the economic policies following from them. I conclude by briefly exploring the viability of a caring economic system in the context of economic globalization.

Chapter 4 extends care theory into the realm of international relations. Sara Ruddick, Fiona Robinson, and others have explored the implications of care ethics for international relations, but offer little in the way of concrete guidelines for caring for distant others. In the first half of this chapter, I fill out their theories by developing a human rights framework based upon human beings' universal duty to care for others. This framework avoids the central shortcomings of other international rights frameworks, including the Universal Declaration of Human Rights (UDHR), and provides a standard of justice that should be reasonably acceptable to people from diverse cultural and religious backgrounds. The second half of the chapter outlines some specific strategies and policies for enforcing human rights abroad and caring for distant others. In Section 4.4 of this chapter, I discuss the conditions under which care theory might justify the use of military force especially for the sake of humanitarian interventions.

The fifth and final substantive chapter addresses the question of how people can be encouraged to be more sympathetic, compassionate, and caring toward others. This topic is important because the long-term stability of a caring society ultimately depends upon the willingness of people to support and comply with caring institutions and policies. I first offer a brief survey of recent psychological studies on the child-rearing practices that are most likely to foster the development of caring attitudes and behaviors in children. In Section 5.2, I propose a number of family policies that would enable and encourage parents to raise their children in a manner likely to foster the sentiments of sympathy and compassion in them. Drawing on the work of Nancy Chodorow, I next argue that the current gendered division of caring within and outside the family must also be addressed if men, in particular, are to become more positively disposed to caring. I then discuss Nel Noddings's proposal for a more caring educational curriculum, and propose an alternative set of educational reforms. Section 5.5 explores the effects of the media, and especially television, on people's attitudes about caring.

I conclude by reflecting upon some personal reasons why we should care for others. Caring is not only morally obligatory but also one key to a happy life. Individuals regularly point to their caring relationships with others as the most fulfilling aspects of their lives. Caring for others is not all drudgery and toil but often a joyous and deeply meaningful experience. Caring institutions and policies not only make the experience of personal caring more available to all human beings, but also expand this experience to our relations with all other human beings. In this way, they make possible a more satisfying and moral existence for all human beings in both our private and public lives.

# 1

# The Nature of Caring and the Obligation to Care

Caring may be defined most generally as feeling or showing concern for something or someone. While caring for things or objects may have great importance for individuals in their personal lives, the main moral importance of caring comes from feeling or showing concern for living beings, and especially human beings.[1] Caring for human beings, in turn, is usually defined as either a virtue or a practice. When caring is defined as a virtue, the focus is on the inner traits, dispositions, and motivations of the caring person. A person may be said to care for others when he or she has the intention and proper disposition to do them good (Gilligan 1982; Halwani 2003; McLaren 2001; Slote 2001; Walker 1998). When caring is defined as a practice, by contrast, the focus is on a person's external actions and their consequences. A person may be said to care for others when he or she helps them actually to satisfy certain needs or achieve certain goals (Ruddick 1989: 13–14). These two definitions of caring are not entirely opposed. Virtue-based definitions usually acknowledge some role for actions, and practice-based definitions generally recognize some role for internal dispositions and relational virtues. The two approaches nonetheless have different emphases. Virtue-based definitions focus on the internal motivations and intentions of caregivers, while practice-based definitions emphasize external actions and their consequences.

Most recent care theorists have endorsed practice-based definitions of caring over virtue-based definitions (Bubeck 1995; Fineman 2004; Held 1993; Kittay 1999; Noddings 2002; Robinson 1999; Ruddick 1989;

---

[1] Care theory can also be extended to include concern or solicitude for animals. See my article 'Care Ethics and Animal Welfare' (2007).

Sevenhuijsen 1998; Tronto 1993; White 2000). Virginia Held argues that virtue-based definitions are too self-involved and miss the centrality of relations to caring. 'To be a caring person requires more than the right virtues or dispositions. It requires the ability to engage in the practice of care, and the *exercise* of this ability' (Held 2006: 51). Nel Noddings similarly argues that it makes no sense to speak of an action as caring unless it meets with some measure of success (Noddings 1992: 16–17; 2002: 19–21, 30, 42–3). If I accidentally spill the glass of water I am carrying to a thirsty person, I fail to care for him or her despite my good intentions. Virtue-based definitions of caring can also offer only limited guidance in developing a political theory. One might use a virtue-based ethic to outline a theory of a caring legislator, statesperson, or social activist, but it is difficult to see how an institution or law could be said to be caring in this motivational sense. In *Morals from Motives*, Michael Slote nonetheless claims it is possible to develop a theory of justice based upon a virtue-based account of caring. One needs only to judge 'customs, laws, and institutions as morally good . . . if they reflect virtuous (enough) motivation on the part of (enough of) those responsible for them and as morally bad (or unjust) if they reflect morally bad or deficient motivation' (2001: 99–100). Slote's theory is innovative and interesting but ultimately difficult to put into practice. Who, after all, should we hold responsible for a particular policy or law (the voters, the legislature, the political party in control of the government?) and how exactly are we to know and judge their motivations?[2] The practice-based approach to care theory is more conducive to developing a general moral and political theory because it identifies actions and goals as definitive of what it means to care.

Most practice-based definitions of caring can be further divided into two general categories: maternalist and generic definitions. Maternalist definitions associate caring with the aims and virtues of ideal mothers or parents (Held 1993; Noddings 2002; Ruddick 1989). In *Starting at Home* (2002), Nel Noddings outlines one of the best developed accounts of this approach to care theory. Rather than starting with a definition of the best state, as philosophers usually do, she begins 'with a description of best homes and then move[s] outward to the larger society' (1). Drawing upon the work of Sara Ruddick (1989), she identifies the central goals

---

[2] Slote addresses this problem in part by specifying a number of objective policies that a caring person or government would support, such as religious toleration and civil freedoms. In specifying these policies, however, Slote seems to shift toward a practice-based account of caring.

of maternal caring as preserving life, promoting growth, and achieving acceptability (Noddings 2002: 176–206). 'The best homes everywhere maintain relations of care and trust, do something to control encounters, provide protection, promote growth, and shape their members in the direction of acceptability' (2002: 123). Noddings then uses this definition of caring to offer suggestions for reforming a number of social policies including housing policy, drug treatment, and abortion (as discussed in Chapter 2).

Since most people intuitively think of parenting as the central example of caring, it makes sense to ground a definition of caring in this activity. Yet maternalist definitions face serious limitations as the basis for a general moral and political theory. Philosophers have long argued that the practices of parents and ideal homes are inappropriate models for relations among competent adults and citizens. Aristotle criticized Plato's ideal republic on these grounds, and Marilyn Friedman similarly notes, 'Morally competent adults, in relationships with each other, do not usually have motherlike responsibilities for each other's preservation, growth, or social acceptability' (Friedman 1993: 151; see also Aristotle 1995: 39–40, 1261a; Dietz 1985; Grimshaw 1986: 249–53). Maternal or parental definitions of caring are also usually (or perhaps unavoidably) rooted in the particular beliefs of groups and cultures about good parenting practices and the nature of the good life, and consequently, tend to be too narrow to support a general moral and political theory (Harris 1991; Hays 1996; Kurtz 1992; Scheper-Hughes 1992: 340–99). Sharon Hays observes that the universal requirements of parenting are fairly minimal, encompassing only those activities necessary to ensure the survival and basic development of the child. 'Beyond these minimal requirements, the methods of child rearing that will best serve the needs of children are ... ambiguous. Although some would argue that current methods of child rearing are the right methods or the most effective methods for preparing children for contemporary society, others would disagree' (Hays 1996: 14). Noddings acknowledges this limitation to her theory, explicitly formulating her definition of ideal parenting practices to nurture open, tolerant, and loving individuals suited for life in a Western liberal democracy (Noddings 2002: 123, 205, 229). By tying her definition of caring to a particular conception of the good life, however, she limits its applicability as the basis for a theory of justice. It will appeal only to individuals who already share her commitment to Western liberal democracy and, more specifically, to the sort of open, tolerant, and caring liberal democratic society that she envisions. Her theory thus ultimately begs the question of why people should embrace her vision of the good life for family and the state.

A second approach to caring defines it more broadly in terms of the generic aims and virtues associated with a variety of caring activities. Joan Tronto and Berenice Fisher have proposed the most influential of these definitions:

> On the most general level, we suggest that caring be viewed as a species activity that includes everything that we do to maintain, continue, and repair our "world" so that we can live in it as well as possible. That world includes our bodies, our selves, and our environment, all of which we seek to interweave in a complex, life-sustaining web. (Tronto 1993: 103)

Tronto and Fisher's definition avoids associating caring with any particular family practices or conception of the good life. It is also broad enough to encompass a wide variety of caring activities including parenting, teaching, and medical care, as well as caring relations among adult citizens. The main drawback of their definition is that it is too broad to guide the development of a moral and political theory. Since much of what we do every day aims in one way or another at maintaining, continuing, or repairing our world, caring is indistinguishable in their definition from many other practices that are not usually considered caring, including housebuilding, plumbing, farming, and so forth.[3] When so broadly defined, caring cannot provide clear recommendations about what we should or should not do morally and politically or where we should place our priorities. Any activity that maintains, continues, or repairs our world can be justified as a form of caring.

In this chapter, I outline a definition of caring that cuts a middle ground between these definitions and provides a more adequate grounding for a general moral and political theory. My definition is guided by two general criteria. First, a good definition of caring should describe the aims and virtues of this practice in a way that encompasses a wide variety of activities that we usually associate with caring, including parenting, teaching, tending to the sick, counseling, and so forth, while excluding all those activities that we usually do not think of as caring, such as plumbing, factory work, music playing, book keeping, and the like. Second, a good definition should describe the aims and virtues of caring across a wide variety of groups, societies, and cultures rather than reflecting the particular aims and virtues of some particular groups or cultures.

---

[3] Fisher and Tronto explicitly designate housebuilding as a form of caring activity (1990: 40).

These two criteria arise from both analytical and political considerations. Analytically, a good definition should aim to describe as many particular instances of a general category as possible, while distinguishing as clearly as possible one category from others. Politically, a good definition should aim to be reasonably acceptable to as many people as possible. Only so can it form the basis of a general conception of justice that all people can reasonably accept.[4]

Section 1.1 of this chapter outlines a definition of caring that fulfills these criteria. In Section 1.2 of the chapter, I develop a theory of obligation for caring that explains why we should care for others. Annette Baier (1994), Martha Fineman (2004), Eva Kittay (1999), and Marilyn Friedman (1993) have all outlined partial theories of obligation for caring. Building upon their arguments, I suggest a fuller theory of obligation based upon my definition of caring. My argument here is Kantian and rationalistic in form but departs from Kant in grounding our duties to others in human interdependency rather than individual autonomy. Moreover, in contrast to most Kantian theories, my theory reserves an important place for emotions, particularity, and partiality in moral action. Section 1.3 of the chapter describes the rightful distribution of our caring responsibilities.

The argument of this chapter provides the moral foundation for the rest of the book, but has value beyond that. My central claim is that caring represents a basic morality for the minimally decent treatment of others that we all should follow. I am not then just laying out the first step of an argument, but also making a general claim about what it means to be a minimally moral person. We should all take seriously our duty to care for others and reflect more deeply upon it, for I am suggesting that caring is at the heart of any cogent account of human morality and justice.

BOTH!  ———————➤  VIRTUES OF CARE
concentrated w/ inner traits

## 1.1. The Definition of Caring

A practice is a general form of activity that can be distinguished from other activities by its distinctive aims, virtues, and sentiments (Ruddick 1989, 13–14). Sculpting, for example, is marked off from other practices by the goal of making a three-dimensional artistic object, and requires a special set of skills and sentiments in order to be performed successfully. Caring as a practice can be distinguished from other activities in a similar fashion. When we care for individuals, we aim to achieve

---

[4] This general notion of morality is defended by Habermas (1990), Rawls (1996), Scanlon (1998), and others.

Care as a practice: distinctive aims?

certain distinctive aims, and if we are to be successful, we must exhibit certain virtues and possess certain sentiments. In this chapter, I discuss primarily the aims and virtues of caring. In Chapter 5, I more fully discuss the disposition to care, including the sentiments of sympathy and compassion and a positive orientation toward caring practices.

While different care theorists have defined the aims of caring in a variety of different ways, most agree that caring at a minimum involves meeting the basic needs of individuals, developing their capabilities, and helping them to survive and function. My own account of the aims of caring clarifies and systematizes this minimalist definition.

When we care for individuals, we most basically help them to satisfy their vital biological needs. Following David Wiggins, vital needs may be defined as those needs that must be met if human beings are to avoid harm or death or having their lives blighted (Wiggins 1998: 6–11). Vital biological needs thus include access to adequate food, sanitary water, appropriate clothing and shelter, sufficient rest, a clean environment, basic medical care, and protection from harm, as well as the need at least among infants and children for physical contact and holding (on this last point, see Bowlby 1969; Winnicott 1965: 37–55). Sexual activity may also be considered a biological need of human beings, but falls outside the scope of caring on the grounds that it is not essential to survival and functioning in the same way that food, water, or medical care are.[5] Since different individuals and groups may manifest their needs for food, clothing, medical care, and other basic goods differently, an important virtue of caring (as discussed below) is meeting individuals' needs according to their particular circumstances and tastes. Since some individuals may require more of some types of goods in order to achieve social functioning, caring also means adjusting the provision of goods to the particular needs of different individuals. In general, though, caring practices may be said to encompass everything we do directly to help individuals to satisfy their vital biological needs so that they can survive, develop, and function.

A second aim of caring is helping individuals to develop or sustain their basic capabilities for sensation, movement, emotion, imagination, reason, speech, affiliation, and in most societies today, literacy and numeracy. The goal here is to enable individuals to develop and maintain as much as

---

[5] Some studies have found correlations between an active sex life and good health, but sex would seem in this regard less a basic prerequisite for survival and functioning and more akin to exercise or activities that people may or may not choose to engage in based upon their vision of the good life.

possible the innate capabilities that are necessary for social functioning, where social functioning means being able to work and obtain the resources necessary for survival, being able to care for oneself and others, and having the opportunity to pursue some conception of the good life. In an earlier article, I argued for a broader understanding of caring, suggesting that it entails fostering the full range of human capabilities described by Martha Nussbaum and John Finnis in their capabilities and natural law theories (Engster 2004). Nussbaum and Finnis include in their lists of human capabilities or basic values a variety of goods such as aesthetic appreciation and expression, religious worship, the pursuit of knowledge, play, friendship, the enjoyment of nature, and political participation (Finnis 1980: 86–90; Nussbaum 2000: 78–80). I now regard my earlier position as mistaken on the grounds that it too closely associates caring with a particular liberal understanding of the good life. If caring is said to involve fostering *all* of the potential capabilities of human beings, then individuals who do not encourage the development of all of these capabilities in their children or others would have to be judged as uncaring. Parents who, for example, meet all their children's biological and basic developmental needs but perhaps for religious reasons choose not to encourage their aesthetic appreciation would be uncaring. Likewise, parents who meet all their children's biological and basic developmental needs but fail to encourage their religious capabilities would also be uncaring. It seems wrong to judge either of these parents as uncaring since, by their own visions of the good life, each may be said to be raising their children in highly caring ways. To say that caring necessarily involves fostering all of a child's complex capabilities ties it too closely to one ideal of a truly human life (Okin 2003).

Based upon these considerations, I now think that caring is better understood in a more basic way, as helping individuals to develop and sustain their *basic or innate capabilities*, including the abilities for sensation, movement, emotion, imagination, reason, speech, affiliation, and in most societies today, the ability to read, write, and perform basic math. These basic capabilities comprise what Nussbaum calls 'the innate equipment of individuals that is the necessary basis for developing the more advanced capabilities, and a ground of moral concern' (Nussbaum 2000: 84). They are more basic than John Rawls's list of primary goods, which includes 'rights and liberties, opportunities and powers, income and wealth' and 'self-respect' (Rawls 1999b: 79, 386). Nonetheless, like Rawls's primary goods, the basic capabilities are goods that we can assume all individuals want whatever else they may want since they are necessary for social

*[handwritten margin note: not just a basic human life form]*

*[handwritten note at bottom: emotional attachment isn't necessary to be caring]*

functioning and underlie the pursuit of any conception of the good life. When parents choose to foster their children's complex capabilities for religion, art, sports, and the like, they may be said to be doing something other than caring for them (which is not to say their actions are uncaring). They are introducing their children to a particular form of the good life.[6]

The third aim of caring is helping individuals to avoid harm and relieve unnecessary or unwanted suffering and pain so that they can carry on with their lives as well as possible. In many cases, this third aim may overlap with the first two, but there may be instances when alleviating pain or suffering has no direct relation to meeting needs or fostering capabilities. As such, this aim stands apart from the other two. The goal here is nonetheless consistent with the other two goals: to enable individuals to carry on with their lives and function in society as much as possible without physical impediments.

As noted above, different individuals may require different types of care and different bundles of goods in order to satisfy their vital biological needs, develop and sustain their innate capabilities, and avoid or alleviate pain and suffering. Individual needs vary, for example, according to age, health, and abilities (Goodin 1995: 244–61; Solomon 1995, 186–93; Wiggins 1998: 11–14). Definitions of adequate clothing or shelter likewise depend on where a person lives and social norms. Different cultures and groups may further define the standards of adequate caring differently. This cultural variability, in particular, raises difficult questions about the nature of caring that I return to discuss below.[7] Standards of minimally adequate care are nonetheless not entirely relative. The ultimate aim of caring is to help individuals to survive, develop, and function in society so that they can care for themselves and others as much as possible and pursue some conception of a good life. As such, caring means at a minimum supporting lives free from malnutrition, illness, exhaustion, and physical danger. It means fostering the greater or lesser basic capabilities of individuals so that they can function as much as possible in society. It means helping individuals to avoid or alleviate pain and suffering whenever possible so that they can carry on with their lives. Altogether, then, caring may be defined as *everything we do directly to help individuals*

[6] Some of these activities, of course, may be useful in helping children to develop their basic or innate capabilities. Parents might choose to enroll their children in a sports league, e.g., to help them develop their physical, emotional, and social capabilities. Insofar as the goal becomes one of honing their children's particular skills or aptitudes in a particular sport, however, then the activity comes to serve ends other than those of caring.

[7] Disagreements that may arise over definitions of adequate caring will be addressed in the discussion of multiculturalism in Chapters 2 and 4.

SURVIVE
DEVELOP
FUNCTION

*to meet their vital biological needs, develop or maintain their basic capabilities, and avoid or alleviate unnecessary or unwanted pain and suffering, so that they can survive, develop, and function in society.* The functional aim of caring provides a standard for judging the adequacy of care in any particular context.[8]

Since caring means *directly* helping a person to meet his or her biological or developmental needs, it may be distinguished from other practices that aim directly at other ends (knowledge, salvation, aesthetic appreciation, and the enjoyment of nature) as well as most forms of productive economic activity. Most economic pursuits are primarily concerned with producing, distributing, and selling goods but not with caring for individuals (Schwarzenbach 1987). The proximate aims of these activities are producing, distributing, and selling commodities, and perhaps most fundamentally in capitalist economies, making money. One may produce a house, shirt, or hamburger for sale but it is usually the person who purchases these goods who uses them for caring. Indeed, one cannot be sure that any commodity will be used to satisfy a biological or developmental need until a person purchases it and actually applies it to this purpose. Caring practices, by contrast, aim directly at helping individuals to satisfy their biological and developmental needs.[9] The crucial question in deciding whether an action is caring is: Can the action be successfully completed without satisfying the biological and developmental needs of a person? A cook in a restaurant can successfully complete the action of making and selling a meal without necessarily caring for anyone. A parent cannot successfully complete the action of nourishing his or her children, however, without making sure that they ingest adequate amounts of nourishing food.

Caring and productive economic activities nonetheless do overlap in one broad occupational area: the caring professions including doctors,

---

[8] In an email correspondence, Nancy Folbre asked: Is baking a birthday cake for a child a form of caring? I would be inclined to say in most cases, yes. In baking a birthday cake for a child or celebrating his or her birthday, we help to develop the child's emotional and social capabilities. We convey to the child a sense that he or she is loved and model the activity of caring for others. By contrast, leaving a store bought cake on the counter for a child with a brief note wishing him or her happy birthday might be deemed uncaring insofar as it conveys to the child an opposite message. The framework outlined here can, I think, be used effectively to judge whether a wide variety of particular actions are caring, but the final assessment will usually depend upon a number of circumstantial considerations.

[9] Here and elsewhere in the remainder of this book, I use the shorthand expressions 'biological and developmental needs' or 'survive, develop, and function' to refer to the aims of caring. The full aims of caring also include helping individuals to sustain their basic capabilities and avoid or alleviate unnecessary or unwanted suffering or pain, but including these elements in every description of the aims of caring becomes unwieldy.

nurses, teachers, childcare workers, counselors, and others. When one pays for the services of these individuals, one purchases their direct care rather than a discrete commodity that may or may not be used for caring. The distinction between caring and noncaring activities is thus emphatically not a distinction between paid and unpaid work, but depends upon the nature of the activity itself. Caring activities include those practices that have as their direct or proximate aims helping individuals to satisfy their biological and developmental needs and avoid or alleviate pain and suffering.

Caring as a practice involves not only satisfying the three basic aims outlined above but also acting according to the virtues of caring. The virtues of caring are those qualities that are necessary for effectively meeting the aims of caring. They are constitutive of caring in the sense that one cannot successfully achieve the aims of caring, or at least cannot do so with any regularity, without them. While care theorists have defined the aims of caring quite differently, there is a good deal of agreement about its core virtues (Noddings 1984, 2002; Tronto 1993).

The first virtue of caring is attentiveness. Lawrence Blum also calls this quality 'moral perception', and defines it as sensitivity to situations that call for a moral response (Blum 1994: 30–61). Attentiveness means noticing when another person is in need and responding appropriately. It also usually involves an ability to anticipate additional needs that a person might have. If an individual is not attentive to others, he or she might meet their most obvious needs but overlook underlying ones—providing them with medication, for example, but failing to cover them with a blanket to keep them warm while they sleep (Blum 1994: 34–6). Most generally, without attentiveness, our caring will be limited or ineffective because we will fail to notice when others are in need or will respond in partial or inappropriate ways (Tronto 1993: 127). Attentiveness most basically directs us to ask the question: Do you need something?

The second virtue of caring is responsiveness. Responsiveness means engaging with others to discern the precise nature of their needs and monitoring their responses to our care (whether verbal or nonverbal) to make sure they are receiving the care they actually need. An individual who fails to engage with others when providing care for them, or fails to monitor their reactions to the care, will in the end usually be less effective than someone who remains open and responsive to them. Noddings notes, for example, that some years ago after a devastating earthquake in Afghanistan, wealthy nations flooded the country with food and clothing when what was needed were building materials (Noddings 2002: 58). The lack of responsiveness in this case made the relief effort less than fully caring. Responsiveness directs us to ask the question: What do you need?

A third virtue of caring is respect. By respect, I do not mean anything so strong as equal recognition of others but more simply the recognition that others are worthy of our attention and responsiveness, are presumed capable of understanding and expressing their needs, and are not lesser beings just because they have needs they cannot meet on their own. One respects others in this sense by treating them in ways that do not degrade them in their own eyes or the eyes of others, and makes use of the abilities they have. While respect might seem to have little to do with actually meeting the needs of others, Julie White has shown otherwise (White 2000). Social service programs that fail to treat their clients with respect tend to breed resentment and mistrust and are less effective than programs that treat their clients as knowledgeable and capable persons. Indeed, people have been known to die or suffer terrible hardships rather than submit to humiliating conditions in order to satisfy their basic needs. Respect directs us to ask the question: What can I do to help you, or even better, what would help you to be able better to meet your needs?

In sum, caring may be said to include everything we do directly to help others to meet their vital biological needs, develop or maintain their innate capabilities, and alleviate unnecessary pain and suffering *in an attentive, responsive, and respectful manner.* The last part of this defin- *goal* ition is important. Caring does not mean thrusting goods at individuals according to what we think they need, but attending and responding to individual needs in respectful ways. In defining caring in this twofold way, my definition may be said to represent a synthesis between what Margaret Urban Walker calls the 'theoretical-juridical model' of morality and the 'expressive-collaborative model' (Walker 1998: 49–75). The theoretical-juridical model defines morality in terms of general rules, aims, or guide-lines that determine what should be done. The expressive-collaborative model relies upon 'a continuing negotiation among people' to reach moral understandings (60). Caring, as I see it, shares elements of both models. Consistent with the theoretical-juridical model, caring aims to satisfy a set of fairly clearly defined goals. In line with the collaborative-expressive model, however, it aims to meet these goals in attentive, respon-sive, and respectful ways. The virtues of attentiveness, responsiveness, and respect importantly distinguish the practice of caring from various pater-nalistic or colonial practices that sometimes masquerade as care (Narayan 1995; White 2000: 123–52). It hardly counts as caring, for example, to give baby formula to poor mothers without consulting them about their

20

needs. Instead, caring requires that we engage in dialogue with others to determine what resources they already have and what we might do to help them. This emphasis on attentiveness, responsiveness, and respect nonetheless need not limit the scope of caring, as care theorists have sometimes suggested (Noddings 1984). We can still care for people across the world; but to care effectively we must be attentive, responsive, and respectful toward them, and avoid treating their needs as self-evident (Tronto 1993: 138).

While caring has thus far been defined as an other-oriented activity, care of self also finds an important place within it (Friedman 1993: 155–63; Gilligan 1982: 128–50, 165; Slote 2001: 77–8; Tronto 1993: 103). We all have biological and developmental needs that must be satisfied if we are to continue to live and function, and meeting these needs represents a form of caring no matter who does it. When we nourish ourselves or take some time to rest, we engage in a caring activity. Caring need not always involve another person. A person who cares only for himself or herself is, of course, usually viewed as selfish rather than caring, and my argument supports this judgment. As I argue below, we all have moral duties to care for others in need when we are able to do so. Nonetheless, caring for oneself is an important form of caring that precedes and in many cases even trumps caring for others (Bubeck 1995: 176–8; Friedman 1993: 155–63; Held 2006: 54–6, 135). Caregivers who do not care for themselves may in the long run be less able or willing to care for others, and further leave themselves open to exploitation and abuse (Held 2006: 135, 138). As Carol Gilligan argued in her foundational work on care theory, a mature care ethic includes an important place for care of self (1982).

The account of caring outlined here fulfills the two definitional criteria stipulated at the beginning of the chapter. First, it captures the central aims and virtues of a variety of activities that we commonly associate with caring, including parenting, teaching, medical care, elder care, counseling, and the like. All these activities aim primarily to meet vital biological and developmental needs of individuals or alleviate pain and suffering. This definition is also narrow enough to exclude practices that may help 'to maintain, continue, and repair our "world"' but are not usually associated with caring, such as housebuilding and plumbing. Housebuilding and plumbing have their own proximate aims that are not necessarily concerned with directly helping individuals to meet their biological and developmental needs. The distinction between caring and noncaring activities is not, of course, absolute. Activities such as housebuilding and plumbing can sometimes be practiced in a caring

Caring of individual self

manner, as when a group of people come together for the explicit purpose of building houses for the homeless. But this activity is then caring only because it is encompassed by a larger caring aim. It is not the activity per se that classifies it as caring or not but its aim and virtues. An activity can be defined as more or less caring to the extent that it more or less directly aims at helping individuals to satisfy their biological needs, develop or maintain their basic capabilities, or avoid or alleviate pain in attentive, responsive, and respectful ways. Plumbing and housebuilding are not usually considered caring because they are most often performed for the direct purpose of transforming the physical world and making money (which, in turn, may or may not be put to caring ends).

The definition of caring outlined here also avoids the cultural, racial, and other biases that limit other definitions. Caring practices admittedly do vary quite a bit among different groups. In non-Western cultures, for example, women tend to maintain closer proximity to their infants and children, sleep more often with them, breastfeed longer, and rely more heavily on communal care arrangements than most Western women (Bhavnagri and Gonzalez-Mena 1997; Garbarino and Ebata 1983; Goldberg 1977; Konner 1977; Korbin 1977, 1979, 1981, 1982; Levine 1977; Sambasivan 2001). Patricia Hill Collins similarly notes that African-Americans tend to rely more heavily upon more communal forms of caring than most middle-class white Americans (Collins 2000). The general definition of caring offered above is nonetheless broad enough to encompass this diversity. It does not identify any specific requirements for how caring must be performed, but instead focuses on the general aims and virtues of caring. Caring is defined as everything people do directly to help others to meet their basic biological needs, develop and maintain their basic capabilities, and alleviate pain and suffering so that they can survive and function in society. All cultures and groups necessarily have practices that match this general definition of caring. If they did not, they could not continue to exist and reproduce themselves. Indeed, researchers who have studied caring practices across cultures have concluded that the differences in forms of caring are relatively trivial compared to their common structural elements (Levine 1977; Lewis and Ban 1977). Despite variations in mothering practices, for example, all infants require attentive, responsive, and respectful caretakers to help them meet their basic needs and foster their development (Hrdy 1999: 96). These common structural elements of caring are not accidental but arise from the common biological and developmental needs of human beings. Human beings would either not survive or develop as similarly as we do across cultures if caring were radically variable. The functional definition of caring offered here can thus lay claim to universality because it associates caring with the generic nurturing activities that all people, cultures, and societies need for their survival and reproduction. Whatever people do to help individuals satisfy their vital biological and developmental needs, and however they do it, may be defined as caring.

Two other factors are often said to be definitive of caring. Many care theorists suggest that emotional engagement or connection is essential in caring for another person (see, e.g. Himmelweit 1999). If the claim here is that emotions such as sympathy and compassion are usually necessary to motivate caring, then it seems right. If the claim is that a person's particular affection for another can sometimes help to improve the quality of their caring, then it also seems correct. However, if the claim is that a person must feel special affection for others in order to care effectively for them, then it seems misguided. It is easy to generate examples of effective caring that involve no special affection for another person. If I pluck a stranger's drowning child from a swimming pool and resuscitate him or her, then I have effectively cared for him or her despite a lack of personal affection. Similarly, if a brusque but competent doctor quickly and accurately sizes up my malady and prescribes medicine for me, he or she has cared for me apparently without, once again, feeling any particular affection for me. Indeed, the idea that emotional affection is inherent to caring practices appears to be rooted in a particularly Western and sentimentalized ideal of caring relationships. Stanley Kurtz notes, for example, that a group of Hindi mothers whom he studied often displayed emotional detachment toward their children in order to foster in them a less individualistic and more collectivistic manner of relating to others in the group (1992: 260–1; see also Sambasivan 2001). Most of these mothers were nonetheless quite effective caregivers. Emotional attachment, then, does not appear to be necessary for effective caring.

Some care theorists further argue that activities should be considered caring only when they help and support 'persons who according to generally accepted social norms . . . cannot take care of themselves' (Bubeck 1995: 129; Schwarzenbach 1987: 155; Tronto 1998; Waerness 1984: 71). Kari Waerness, in particular, draws a distinction between necessary care and personal services, and excludes from her definition of caregiving all personal services such as making dinner for individuals who are capable of performing this task themselves (Waerness 1984). This distinction is important because it separates out those cases where individuals are truly in need of care from those where care is trivial, or more sinisterly, where one party holds power over another and compels the other to serve him or her. Nonetheless, it seems problematic to define away all cases of personal service as noncaring. If caring can only be said to occur when one party satisfies some need that another cannot reasonably satisfy on his or her own, then most cases of everyday caring among adults would no longer count as caring. It further seems strange to define a practice according to the neediness of the person toward whom it is directed. We do not usually define flute playing or book keeping in these terms, so why caring? The definition of caring offered here makes no distinction between necessary care and personal services. We care for others whenever we help them to meet their basic or developmental needs or to avoid or alleviate pain. Making dinner for one's capable spouse or partner is an act of caring, just as making dinner for a child or sick friend is. However, as I argue in Section 1.3, we have a moral obligation to care for others only in cases where individuals cannot reasonably meet their needs on their own. Personal service care, as Waerness defines it, is thus not morally obligatory.

Based upon this definition of caring, there are at least three distinct ways to care for others. First, one may personally care for others by meeting their needs, fostering their basic capabilities, or alleviating their pain or suffering in an attentive, responsive, and respectful manner. Personal care is the paradigmatic case of caring, and may also include supervising and financially supporting an individual's personal care, as when a parent takes his or her child to a doctor (Kittay, Jennings, and Wasunna 2005: 444). Second, one may care for others by providing their caregivers with the resources and support necessary to provide good care for them. Eva Kittay has dubbed this form of caregiving *doulia* after the postpartum caregiver, the doula, who cares for the mother so that she can better care for her child (Kittay 1999: 106–7). This form of caring is less personal than the paradigm case, but still fits the definition of caring because the direct aim of the activity remains meeting the needs and fostering the capabilities of others—in this case, of both caregiver and care-receiver.[10] Third, one may care for others collectively by supporting institutions and policies that directly help individuals to meet

---

[10] 'Doulia' is similar to 'provisioning', or the act of directly providing the goods or resources necessary for caring (Nelson 1993). While doulia or provisioning is an important form of caring, it is usually not sufficient in close relationships. Individuals in close relationships usually have more needs than can be met simply by providing resources for them. Thus, a person who cares for his family (as men sometimes do) solely through provisioning is only minimally (and usually deficiently) caring toward them.

their needs, develop or sustain their basic capabilities, or live as much as possible free from pain and suffering (e.g. public housing programs, public education programs, public health programs). In collective caring, our contribution is smaller and more diffuse, but still counts as caring insofar as the direct aim remains helping individuals to meet their biological and developmental needs in attentive, responsive, and respectful ways. Government agencies or community service organizations serve as our agents (or as doulas) in collective caring by actually providing care to individuals. We contribute to the care of others in this most general or collective sense by promoting, supporting, and complying with governmental institutions and policies that directly support and accommodate caring practices.[11]

## 1.2. The Obligation to Care

Having defined the nature of caring in Section 1.1, I now turn to develop a rational account of our obligation to care for others. The purpose is to explain why we should care for others in need when we are able to do so. Care theorists have often looked upon rational justifications for caring with some skepticism (Donovan 1996; Luke 1996; Noddings 1984; Robinson 1999). For these theorists, the motivation to care for others is rooted in emotions such as sympathy and compassion. By their account, one either feels sympathy and compassion for others or one does not, and there seems to be little point in arguing with someone who does not already recognize caring for others as a moral good (Warren 2000: 112–13). In setting forth a theory of obligation for caring, I do not mean to deny the important role that sympathy and compassion play in motivating and facilitating caring practices. A person lacking in sympathy and compassion would have to struggle constantly to stay motivated to care for others and remain attentive and responsive to their needs. Even so, a theory of obligation can play an important role within care theory in a number of ways.

As noted in the Introduction, even if human beings are born with a natural proclivity for sympathy and compassion, these emotions still need to be cultivated. When children are not encouraged to develop sympathy and compassion, they usually do not grow up with a strong sense of concern for others. If we think it important that individuals should feel

---

[11] This idea of collective caring is further discussed in Chapter 2.

sympathy and compassion for others, we should therefore try to organize our social practices, policies, and institutions to facilitate the development of these sentiments. The question then arises: why should we organize our social practices, policies, and institutions to support these sentiments rather than some others? A theory of obligation offers an answer to this question. By showing that we have a moral obligation to care for others, it demonstrates that we should organize our social policies, practices, and institutions to support the development of sympathy and compassion because these sentiments are crucial for motivating moral behavior. Without a rational defense for caring, it is at least not self-evident why people should encourage the development of sympathy and compassion rather than, say, competitiveness and egoism.

A rational theory of obligation can also be useful in explaining why we should extend our sympathy and care to individuals outside our immediate social circle. As even most care theorists acknowledge, many people's natural sympathies are weak when it comes to caring for others outside their immediate family and friends. Nationalists, racists, and others may feel great sympathy and compassion for individuals within their group but contempt for individuals outside it. Care theorists are then faced with the question of explaining why we *should* care for strangers and distant others. A rational theory of obligation is important for answering this question. By demonstrating that we should care for all human beings, it can correct for parochial applications of our sympathy and compassion and challenge ideologies that may constrict the scope of these emotions.[12]

A rational theory of obligation can further play some role in developing or strengthening our sentiments of sympathy and compassion. When care theorists reject rationalist theories of obligation, they effectively reinforce the traditional Western framework that pits reason against emotion in moral thinking. Instead of privileging reason over emotion, as Western philosophers usually have done, they simply privilege the emotions over the reason. Yet, they continue to treat reason and emotion as separate, and in some sense incompatible, modes of moral thinking. Robert Solomon, Martha Nussbaum, and others have argued, by contrast, that the long-standing dichotomy between reason and emotion is misguided

---

[12] Hume argued in this regard that reason can correct 'the inequalities of our internal emotions and perceptions' (Hume [1751] 1983: 48). Martha Nussbaum similarly notes that compassion 'needs a correct view of the people who should be the objects of our concern' to guard against parochialism and avoid reinforcing 'hierarchies of class, race, and gender' (Nussbaum 2001: 387).

(Damasio 1994; Nussbaum 2001; Solomon 1995). The emotions are not untamed impulses without any relation to our thoughts and reason but contain important cognitive elements. They are, to paraphrase Nussbaum and Solomon, forms of evaluative judgment that ascribe some value or importance to certain things and persons for an individual's sense of identity, well-being, or goals (Nussbaum 2001: 22–23; Solomon 1995: 220).[13] They alert us in an intuitive way, and usually before our reason can react, to situations that should concern us. We feel fear or anxiety when we perceive a threat to our lives and well-being. We feel anger or sadness when someone whose life and well-being we consider integral to our own happiness is harmed or becomes sick.

Because emotions contain a cognitive element, they can be at least partially transformed through rational reflection (Nussbaum 2001: 232–3; Solomon 1995: 222–3).[14] Indeed, what we feel and whom we feel for is often shaped by our frame of reference. By reflecting on a perceived threat, for example, and noting that it does not really represent a danger to our lives or well-being, we may be able to lessen our fear or anxiety. A theory of obligation for caring can similarly transform our feelings of sympathy and compassion for others. By reflecting upon our obligation to care for others, we may come to regard the hunger and suffering of others as matters of concern to us affecting our sense of ourselves as moral persons. We may likewise come to see parochial ideologies and other blocks to our sympathy and compassion as immoral. In short, a theory of obligation for caring can help us to develop or strengthen the emotions that motivate us to act in caring ways. In the final analysis, this is perhaps all that any moral theory can do: inspire in us a desire to act morally according to a set of precepts that can be shown rationally to be right.

Some readers may nonetheless remain skeptical about the power of reason to inspire this sort of moral transformation. While a rational theory of obligation might show that we behave inconsistently or contradictorily in not caring for others, an immoralist might wryly respond with a few well-chosen lines from Walt Whitman's 'Song of Myself:'

---

[13] Nussbaum notes some differences between her account of emotions and Solomon's view (22 n. 2).

[14] As most cognitive therapists will readily admit, the process of transforming our emotions through cognitive reflection is usually not an easy or quick one, and there may be limits to the extent to which cognitive reflection can change our emotions. My point here is modest: that we can change at least some of our emotions some of the time through rational reflection.

> Do I contradict myself?
> Very well then I contradict myself;
> (I am large, I contain multitudes). (Whitman 1980: 82)[15]

A person who adopts this position is unlikely to be persuaded by rational arguments, but few people are so glib about their moral beliefs. Once a person gives up even the pretense of attempting to provide some sort of rational account of his or her moral actions and beliefs, he or she forsakes all possibility of moral cooperation with individuals who think differently from him or her. No longer can this person be said to be interested in coordinating his or her actions with others according to generally accepted standards, but only in announcing his or her views and bending others to his or her will. Since most individuals at least wish to think of themselves as moral persons, most people are willing to grant rational arguments at least some influence over their moral views, and some individuals may even be affected by rational arguments at the basic emotional level.

My account of caring, then, includes a place for both emotions and reason. The emotions of sympathy and compassion are important for motivating and facilitating the delivery of care. Reason, however, can guide and expand these sentiments and perhaps even strengthen and develop them. While my argument in this chapter focuses on reasons for caring, I return in Chapter 5 to explore how cultural institutions such as the family and schools can foster the development of sympathy and compassion in people. Both ends of my argument are equally important. Emotion and reason are both necessary for the development and maintenance of caring persons and a caring society.

Not all care theorists are opposed to developing rational justifications of caring. Annette Baier, Eva Kittay, Martha Fineman, and others have outlined some justifications for a duty to care for others (Baier 1994, 1997; Clement 1996; Code 1987b; Fineman 2004; Held 1993; Kittay 1999, 2001).[16] Eva Kittay and Grace Clement, for example, have drawn upon Robert Goodin's vulnerability model to develop a theory of obligation for care ethics (Clement 1996: 73–4; Kittay 1999: 54–73). Goodin begins with the intuition that we all have special moral obligations to family and friends, and suggests that these obligations are best explained in terms of these individuals' vulnerability to our actions and choices (Goodin

---

[15] On this critique of rational obligation, see Noddings (2002: 113–14).

[16] Nancy Hirschmann has outlined a feminist theory of obligation that relates more to questions of political obligation generally (Hirschmann 1992).

1985). Because our family and friends are especially vulnerable to our actions and choices, he claims we have special responsibilities to look out for their welfare. Goodin then extends this model to encompass our relations with fellow citizens and strangers in foreign countries. If we have moral obligations to family and friends because they are vulnerable to us, we must also have moral obligations to fellow citizens and distant strangers, since they are in many cases likewise vulnerable to our actions and choices. These obligations include not only the negative duty to refrain from causing them harm but also the positive duty to meet their needs when we are in position to do so (Goodin 1985: 110–11).

Although Goodin's argument is not meant to provide a normative ground for care theory, Kittay and Clement have applied it to this purpose, arguing that a duty to care for others can be derived from their vulnerability to us. There is a problem, however, with using Goodin's argument in this way. Goodin does not actually provide an account of why we should care about the interests or vulnerability of others, but merely assumes this point. He starts out with the widely held moral intuition that we have special obligations to our family and friends, explains these obligations in terms of their vulnerability to us, and concludes that we must also have moral obligations to distant others because they are similarly vulnerable to our actions. Nowhere, though, does he explain why we should care about the interests or vulnerability of our family and friends. He assumes the very thing care theorists wish to demonstrate: that we should care about the needs of others.

The vulnerability of others does not in fact generate a duty to care for them. There is nothing about vulnerability per se that obligates a caring response. At the very least, some further argument is necessary in order to show why vulnerability should generate an obligation to care. Baier, Kittay, and Fineman have all partially developed alternative theories of obligation based upon our dependency on others (Baier 1994, 1997; Fineman 2004; Kittay 2001). When further extended and clarified, this dependency approach offers a far more persuasive justification for our duty to care. We may all be said to have obligations to care for others not so much because others are vulnerable to us, but rather because we are (and have been and will be) dependent upon others. It is our dependency on others rather than their vulnerability to us that ultimately grounds our obligation to care for them.

Our dependency on others for caring takes a variety of forms. Most obviously, all human beings require care during childhood to survive and develop their capabilities. Infants and small children would not survive for very long or develop the basic capabilities necessary to survive without the care of some sort of parenting figure or figures (Code 1987*b*). In fact, human beings are far more dependent upon care—both in terms of quantity and quality—than our nearest genetic relatives (Hrdy 1999: 267–9). Human infants depend upon their caretakers for food and protection longer than any of the apes, and also require much more attention and training to develop their sensory, motor, emotional, linguistic, and reasoning abilities. In this respect, Baier has suggested that what makes us human, at least as much as anything else, is the care we receive from other humans. 'A person, perhaps, is best seen as one who was long enough dependent upon other persons to acquire the essential arts of personhood. Persons essentially are second persons, who grow up with other persons' (Baier 1985: 84). We develop the capabilities necessary for what most people consider a minimally decent human life, including our emotions, language, reasoning, and sociability, through the care of other human beings. Children raised in the wild without human care, even when they are able to survive, never develop the basic emotional, linguistic, reasoning, and other capabilities that greatly facilitate survival and are necessary for living with others in society (Code 1987*a*: 171).[17]

We do not simply graduate once and for all from a state of childhood dependency to full adult independence, but further require caring throughout our lives for our survival and basic functioning. Fineman and Kittay note that 'early childhood, illness, disability and frail old age' are not exceptional circumstances in our lives but 'inevitable dependencies' rooted in our biology (Fineman 1995: 161–2; Kittay 1999: 29).[18] Alasdair MacIntrye makes a similar point:

We human beings are vulnerable to many kinds of affliction and most of us are at some time afflicted by serious ills. How we cope is only in small part up to us. It is most often to others that we owe our survival, let alone our flourishing, as we encounter bodily illness and injury, inadequate nutrition, mental defect and disturbance, and human aggression and neglect. (MacIntyre 1999: 4)

[17] Mary Midgley further notes, 'Stories of wolf-children, etc. are hard to evaluate, partly because the actual evidence is slight, partly because all have died soon after capture. It seems impossible that a child should be brought up *from the start* by wolves or any other terrestrial species, because the sheer physical work needed is beyond them' (1984: 107).

[18] Ruth O'Brien similarly argues that disability should not be seen as an exceptional condition but rather as in many ways paradigmatic of the human condition: 'disability should not be viewed as an identity, but rather as a condition that shapes how people do things. This condition, moreover, is ever-changing. Few people escape facing it sometime in their lifetime. This is inherent in our organic nature—all people are dying. Hence, the term "disabled" should not be used to characterize the unusual mind or body; it describes what habitually happens to the mind or body. It captures the *human* condition' (O'Brien 2005: 35).

The need for caring is most urgent and obvious during childhood, illness, disability, and old age, but also runs throughout our everyday lives. Even during times of relative health and vigor, most of us look daily to spouses, partners, parents, friends, and associates to help us with cooking, child-care, emotional stress, and other basic life needs, and many of us look to these same individuals to help us through periods of financial or personal hardship. We further look to others for the continuing development and maintenance of many of our basic capabilities. Our basic emotional, imaginative, and reasoning capabilities are not simply and fully developed by childhood's end, but continue to grow and evolve in our relations with others throughout our lives.

Many of us further experience another form of dependency in our lives—the dependency that comes from caring for another (Fineman 2004: 35–7; Kittay 1999: 106–09). Caring for another often means depend-ing upon others for material resources and other forms of support or accommodation. Fineman dubs this form of dependency 'derivative dependency' since it arises from caring for an 'inevitably dependent per-son' (Fineman 2004: 35–6). Yet, for many people, this form of depend-ency is no more avoidable than the inevitable biological dependencies discussed above. Few of us have the abilities or resources to engage in intensive care for another person without in some way depending upon others to help us meet our needs and supply provisions for the care of this person. When we depend upon other people for care, this means that we also are usually dependent upon others beyond just our pri-mary caregivers. We depend upon all those individuals who support or accommodate our caregivers so that they can care for us. Our survival and development ultimately depends upon an extensive web of social relations that makes caring possible.

We finally all depend upon the caring of others to reproduce society and to make civil life possible. If no one cared for others, society would cease to exist within a couple of generations (Kittay 1999: 28, 92). Then our own ability to survive, develop, and receive care from others would be seriously compromised. 'Without aggregate caretaking there could be no society, so we might say that it is caretaking labor that produces and reproduces society' (Fineman 2004: 48). We also all depend upon others to nurture the sorts of human beings capable of social cooperation and making social contributions. 'Caretaking labor provides the citizens, the workers, the voters, the consumers, the students, and others who populate society and its institutions' (Fineman 2004: 48). We thus all depend upon the caring of others *for others* to produce individuals with whom we can become friends, marry, engage in sociable and productive activities, and rely upon if necessary for the care we may need to survive and function. The care of others for others supports the social environment that sustains us.

Given the necessity of caring practices for the maintenance and reproduction of society, Virginia Held highlights the inadequacy of social contract theories that start out by imagining a number of independent and self-sufficient individuals in the state of nature: 'Before there could have been any self-sufficient, independent men in a hypothetical state of nature, there would have to have been mothers and the children these men would have been' (Held 1993: 195). It might be added that these mothers would have had to have been 'good enough' at their care work so that these men could develop the basic capabilities and trust necessary to form a social contract. Nancy Folbre suggests in a similar vein that caring for children ought to be reconceived as a public good, since we all benefit or suffer depending upon the quality of care provided to children:

Parents who raise happy, healthy, and successful children create an especially important public good. Children themselves are not the only beneficiaries. Employers profit from access to productive workers. The elderly benefit from Social Security taxes paid by the younger generation. . . . Fellow citizens gain from having productive and law-abiding neighbors. These are all examples of positive spillovers and side effects that economists often call 'positive externalities' because they are external to the actual decision to provide care. (Folbre 2001: 50)

Folbre's point can be extended to other forms of care as well. The care provided for injured, sick, elderly, or disabled individuals does not just benefit them, but usually has other positive externalities. It enables these individuals to contribute to society when and in whatever ways they can—productive, relational, or other.

There are perhaps other ways in which we are dependent upon others for care, but the preceding arguments should suffice to make the point: we are all unavoidably and deeply dependent upon the care of others. We depend upon others for caring during childhood, sickness, disability, and old age. Most of us depend upon the care of others in our day-to-day lives and during times of particular hardship. We depend upon the care that others give to others to reproduce society, and most caregivers (whose work we depend upon) are dependent upon others to perform their care work. In short, we live in a web of dependency and caring. It is not just that we have depended and probably will depend upon the care of others one day; rather, human existence is inextricably implicated in relations of dependency and caring. Even when we are not immediately dependent upon the personal care of some particular individual, we still depend upon the care of many others for our survival and social functioning.

Pointing to these sorts of dependencies, Fineman argues that 'caretaking work creates a collective or societal debt' that obligates each of us to help support caring activities (Fineman 2004: 47). Accordingly, she argues that we should spread out the costs of caregiving among all its beneficiaries to reflect its broad social value. Kittay likewise suggests that the duty to care for others should be understood as a 'categorical imperative ... derivable from universalizing our own understanding that were we in such a situation, helpless and unable to fend for ourselves, we would need care to survive and thrive' (Kittay 2001: 535). While Fineman's and Kittay's statements are suggestive, neither develops them very fully. In the following pages, I extend their insights by arguing that our inevitable and pervasive dependency on others can generate a theory of obligation for caring. Before outlining this argument, however, I briefly outline two partial, albeit ultimately inadequate, justifications for our duty to care for others.

Most basically, we all have self-interested, or prudential, reasons to care for others. We all need the care of others at some point during our lives, and one effective way to ensure that we all receive quality care when we need it is to set up collective programs to make sure it is available to everyone. By ensuring good care for all individuals in our social environment, we also increase the likelihood that we will be surrounded by more capable and sociable, and fewer incapable and maladjusted, individuals. This, in turn, will enable us to live fuller and safer lives, and increase the probability that the individuals around us will be able to provide us with decent care when we need it. There are nonetheless limitations to this self-interested justification for our caring duties. Prudential considerations would seem to direct us to try to reap the benefits of caring as much as possible while contributing as little as possible to its support. Likewise, if our duty to care rests upon nothing more than self-interest, then we might justifiably isolate ourselves and our loved ones into narrow, resource-rich, caring communities (as some people in fact attempt to do), and neglect all others. Care theorists have generally rejected this understanding of caring on the grounds that it conflicts with intuitive understandings of what it means to be a caring person, and as I argue below, this intuition is right (Card 1990: 102; Tronto 1993: 171).

Annette Baier has suggested that we might overcome these problems by recasting our duty to care for others in terms of the principle of fairness (Baier 1997: 5–7, 29–31). The principle of fairness states that

*[handwritten margin note: self interested: a healthy community better for self]*

*[handwritten margin note: principle of fairness]*

all individuals are obligated to contribute their fair share to the maintenance of any cooperative scheme that mutually benefits them (Klosko 1992; Rawls 1999b; Simmons 1979: 101–42). Baier argues that caring may be understood as such a cooperative scheme. We all depend, or have depended, upon parents, family, friends, spouses, teachers, doctors, nurses, and others for our survival and functioning. We likewise all depend upon the care these figures give, or have given, to others in our social environment for our social existence and well-being. We may therefore all be said to have a duty to contribute our fair share to the cooperative scheme of caring. Baier writes in this regard that 'free riding on the generative scheme' of caring is 'at best churlish, at worst manifestly unjust' since caring forms the background of society and is central to the quality of all of our lives (Baier 1997: 30). To benefit from the caring that others provide or have provided to us and others, and yet to refuse to contribute into the caring scheme, violates the most basic principle of fairness, and ultimately erodes the basic preconditions of human existence and social reproduction.

The principle of fairness provides a broader basis than self-interest for justifying our obligation to care for others, but is still inadequate. First, it limits our caring duties to individuals with whom we share a cooperative scheme. This is not necessarily a fatal flaw, but it does mean that our caring duties will be somewhat parochial. We will have duties to care only for those individuals who in some way exist in our immediate social web. Second, and more disconcertingly, the principle of fairness limits our caring duties only to those individuals capable of contributing to the cooperative scheme of caring. Based upon this principle, severely disabled persons who will never be able to care for others would seem to have no rightful claim to receive care from others since they may never be able to contribute to the care of others (Goodin 1995: 279–80). Even care for infants has to be justified in this theory through the expectation that they will someday care for us or others.

The shortcomings of both the self-interested and fairness accounts of our caring duties can be overcome by formulating a theory of obligation modeled loosely after Alan Gewirth's moral theory (Gewirth 1978, 1996). Gewirth's moral theory employs what he calls the 'dialectically necessary method' to identify our underlying moral commitments (1978: 42–7). The dialectically necessary method does not rely upon the actual beliefs, thoughts, or statements of individuals, but rather draws out the moral claims and principles necessarily implied by people's actions. It thus does not provide a description of what people actually claim or believe morally, but identifies moral principles that follow from the universal necessary features of human existence. While I draw upon Gewirth's methodology, it is important to note that the substance of my argument departs radically from his. Gewirth's argument rests at root upon human autonomy and purposive action; my own is based upon human dependency and the need for care. By rooting my argument in dependency and caring, I not only reach a different set of moral conclusions from Gewirth, but also avoid some of the main problems associated with his argument.[19]

The first step of my argument is as follows: (1) *All human beings can be assumed to value their survival, the development and functioning of their basic capabilities, and the avoidance or alleviation of unwanted pain and suffering—unless they explicitly indicate otherwise.* If individuals did not value these goods, they presumably would not act to satisfy their needs, practice their capabilities, and avoid pain and suffering as we all do every day. Even infants exhibit a variety of activities including clinging, suckling, crying, and fussing that point to an implicit desire to survive and develop the capabilities necessary for survival. The desire for survival, development, and basic functioning can further be inferred among sleeping, unconscious, or incapacitated individuals (unless they have previously indicated otherwise) based upon their prior conscious activities and what we generally know about human behavior.

*desire for survival, development, avoidance*

Now, as indicated above, *(2) all human beings depend upon the care of others to survive, develop and maintain their basic capabilities, and avoid or alleviate unwanted pain and suffering.* As such, *(3) all human beings can be said at least implicitly to value caring as a necessary good and to make claims on others for care when we need it, meaning that we at least implicitly assert that others should help us to meet our basic needs, develop and maintain our basic capabilities, and avoid or alleviate pain when we cannot reasonably achieve these goods on our own.* A person in need of care will generally claim that others should help him or her. The normative content of this claim is supplied by the person in need, and need not (at least at this point in the argument) be recognized as normatively binding on others. The claim is, to borrow the language of Joel Feinberg, aspirational rather than a

---

[19] Martin Golding writes, e.g.: 'Gewirth starts with a philosophically minimal given, the situation of the rational, self-interested agent, and goes on to define philosophically substantial conclusions. I have argued that careful attention to this situation, and to what an agent is committed to, undercuts Gewirth's enterprise. An enriched starting point, stronger philosophical premises, is needed in order to demonstrate the existence of human rights' (Golding 1981: 173). For other criticisms focusing on Gewirth's starting point of autonomous agency, see also Friedman (1981) and Morris (1981). For an extensive discussion of criticisms of Gewirth's theory, and defense of this theory, see Beyleveld (1991).

valid rights claim (Feinberg 1970*b*). The person in need asserts that others *should* help him or her to achieve a set of goods that he or she values and cannot achieve without their help. A person who is being assaulted or drowning will usually call out for help and at least implicitly assert the moral duty of others to help him or her, regardless of how others may view his or her claims. The same may be said of a person who is desperately in need of food or water. Even the demands of infants for care have something of this quality. Since their survival and development depends upon the care of others, they implicitly (or not so implicitly) make strong demands on others to care for them that extend beyond mere pleas for beneficence.[20]

Individuals need not, however, always actually voice or indicate their desire for care in order to make a claim on others. The claim follows necessarily from their desire for survival, development, and functioning, and their need for the care of others to achieve these aims. A claim for care can be inferred, for example, among infantile, incapacitated, comatose, shy, or reserved persons from the very presence of a dire need that they cannot reasonably meet on their own. The language of claiming therefore must be distinguished in this argument from its usual voluntaristic associations. We all claim care from others by virtue of our dependency on them for goods that we all desire. Whether we actually voice or indicate our needs to others is inconsequential, though it does increase the likelihood that our needs will be noticed.

Some individuals may occasionally waive off offers of caring because they (perhaps mistakenly) do not consider themselves truly to be in need, or because they no longer wish to survive, or because they consider some other value such as pride or honor as more important in a particular instance than their survival, development, or functioning. Individuals do always have the right to refuse the care of others. Yet, just because individuals may refuse care in one or another situation does not mean they escape the web of caring relations. All people have sought care from others at some time in their lives (at the very least during infancy), and will be likely to do so again insofar as they value their survival, development, and functioning above other goods. Caring is so integral to our survival, development, and functioning that the desire for any of these goods (which is implied by our daily pursuit of them) implies a desire that others at least offer us care if we should need it.

[20] Martha Nussbaum makes a similar point: 'Any failure on the part of the caretaker to fulfill those wants [of the infant] will lead to reactive anger, as if (to put it in prematurely complex terms) some right of its own had been slighted' (2001: 192).

The fourth step of the argument identifies a general moral principle that is implied by our dependency on others for care: *(4) In claiming care from others, we imply that capable human beings ought to help individuals in need when they are able to do so consistent with their other caring obligations.* In actual practice, individuals may make use of more particular principles to attempt to justify their caring claims, drawing upon familial ties or group loyalties. Individuals are nevertheless necessarily committed to the more general justifying principle outlined above—at least insofar as they value their survival, development, and functioning—for two reasons. First, our needs might be met by any capable human being and we cannot know in advance who might help us. In calling upon others for care, we effectively say: anyone capable of helping me (and others like me with similar needs, if we are to be consistent) ought to care for me. Thus: capable human beings ought to care for human beings in need. If our parents, friends, or compatriots happen to be available, we might bypass this general justification for more particular, conventional, or emotive ones. But the more general justification is always lingering just behind these other justifications. The second reason we are necessarily committed to this general moral principle is because our claims on particular others for care almost always involve others besides them. As argued above, potential caregivers often need the care of others in order to be able to provide care to us. The particular care we seek always exists within a web of linked and nested social relations (Kittay 1999: 66–70). In making claims on others for care in any particular situation, we therefore have to make claims on many others beyond our immediate potential caregivers. At the very least, we usually have to claim caring for our caregivers in claiming care for ourselves. Our own particular claims thus necessarily require claiming and justifying care for anyone in need. Indeed, at the most general level, our particular claims on others for care involve the broad social claim that all capable human beings ought to help all individuals in need, since otherwise society would not exist and there would be no one available to care for us.

There are nonetheless moral limits to the response we might legitimately expect from others. Because our claim for care is justified through a general moral principle, we should be able to understand if individuals forgo helping us when it would involve extreme danger to themselves, seriously compromise their long-term functioning, or impede their ability to care for other individuals. Morally speaking, our own care does not outweigh the care of other individuals, including their care for themselves.

Up to this point in the argument, the moral claims we make upon others for care remain unjustified. We may think it would be a very good thing if others were to care for us in times of need, and may even acknowledge that our claims upon others commit us to the general moral principle discussed above. Yet, there would seem to be no necessary reason why others should satisfy our claims for caring upon them. Their care would always seem to be a gift.

The validation of our claims for care appears in the fifth and final step of the argument. When individuals all needing care from others and making claims upon others for care are placed in a social context of relationships and dependency, then each can validate his or her claims for care on others by appealing to the general moral principle that all individuals have necessarily used in claiming care for themselves. Because all individuals have sought care from others, we all have made use of the general moral principle that capable individuals ought to care for individuals in need. All capable individuals should therefore logically recognize and honor this moral principle when others make use of it to validate their claims for caring on them. Loosely following Gewirth, we may dub this final step in the argument *the principle of consistent dependency:* (5) *Since all human beings depend upon the care of others for our survival, development, and basic functioning and at least implicitly claim that capable individuals should care for individuals in need when they can do so, we should consistently recognize as morally valid the claims that others make upon us for care when they need it, and should endeavor to provide care to them when we are capable of doing so without significant danger to ourselves, seriously compromising our long-term functioning, or undermining our ability to care for others.* Capable individuals who refuse to honor this principle violate the logical principle of noncontradiction and behave hypocrit- ically. They fail to recognize and honor the moral principle that they themselves have made use of (and likely will make use of again one day) to justify their own care. More seriously, they implicitly renounce the web of caring upon which their own lives, society, and human life generally depend.

*b/c we all need care.*

The principle of noncontradiction brings about the transition from a prudential to a moral rights claim for care. An individual in need can rationally justify his or her claim on others for care by pointing out that they have called upon others to care for them and implicitly justified their right to care on the very grounds now being invoked— that capable human beings ought to care for others in need insofar as they are able to do so. There is a circular quality to this argument for our duty to care for others, and intentionally so. Care theory derives our moral obligations not from some abstract moral ground such as autonomy or self-consciousness but rather from our relations with others as dependent social creatures. We have duties to care for others because we have appealed to others for care, and other individuals have duties to us because they have appealed to still others. There might perhaps be some point in the recesses of evolutionary history when the first claim for care was made upon another and satisfied out of sheer benevolence. But here and now, every living human being has made claims on others for care and consequently has obligated himself or herself to help others to meet their biological and developmental needs when and if he or she is able to do so. Our duty to care for others ultimately derives from our nature as dependent creatures who need the care of others to survive, develop, and function.

The principle of consistent dependency is similar to the principle of fairness discussed above, but broader. It grounds our duty to care for others not in relations of reciprocity but in our common human dependency. As such, it does not have the exclusionary implications of the fairness principle. It does not matter for the principle of consistent dependency that severely disabled persons may never be able to care for us or others. We are bound to care for them because they are dependent upon us for their survival and functioning just as we are (and have been and likely will be) dependent on others. We have all made and continue to make claims on others similar to the ones that severely disabled persons make upon us. Indeed, severely disabled persons are not a 'special case' in care theory, as they are in so many moral philosophies, but paradigmatic of the dependency that all human beings experience at various times during our lives (O'Brien 2005).

The principle of consistent dependency is also narrower and more precise than the golden rule. We are not obligated by the principle of consistent dependency to do unto others whatever we would have done to ourselves, but rather to provide them with the care they need to survive and function. Moreover, we must attend and respond to others' needs given their abilities and circumstances instead of projecting onto them our ideas about what we want others to do unto us.

The principle of consistent dependency finally avoids one of the central weaknesses of Gewirth's theory. Gewirth's argument depends upon the willingness of individuals to recognize themselves and others as

50

autonomous agents. Gewirth himself, however, identifies some arbitrary standards for the recognition of autonomous agency. He argues, for example, that animals, children, and mentally impaired individuals are not autonomous agents—even though they apparently engage in all sorts of purposive actions—and thus are not entitled to the full rights of autonomous agents (Gewirth 1978: 119–127, 1996: 24, 65). By his estimation, they lack some essential characteristic of autonomous agency, such as the 'ability to control their behavior by their unforced choice, to have knowledge of relevant circumstances beyond what is present to immediate awareness, and especially to reflect rationally on their purposes' (1978: 120). Racists, sexists, and nationalists have, of course, often reached similar conclusions about people of color, women, and others. They would therefore seem to be no more inconsistent in depriving these groups of full rights than Gewirth is in denying full rights to animals, children, and mentally impaired individuals.

Care theory avoids these problems by rooting our moral obligations to others in our empirically verifiable dependency upon others and others' dependency upon us. While it might be possible to deny the autonomous agency of some individuals based upon their mental capacity, sex, race, ethnicity, or other characteristics, it hardly seems plausible to deny their dependency. Even just refusing to extend caring to others in need involves implicitly acknowledging their dependency upon us. One might nonetheless attempt to deny the duty to care for some others on the ground that they are not really 'human', or lack some special characteristic that individuals must possess in order to be worthy of caring. These sorts of arguments are, however, contradictory. Our own claims for caring do not depend upon any abstract definition of what it means to be human, or any particular attributes that we may possess, but stem from the fact that we are the sort of dependent creatures whose survival, development, and functioning requires the care of certain sorts of creatures (i.e. humans) who are uniquely capable of helping us to achieve these goals. Our own claims for care thus logically commit us to extend care to all other beings who necessarily depend upon human care for their survival, development, and functioning. If another creature meets these criteria, we are logically obligated to care for him or her.[21] Abstract definitions of

---

[21] Other creatures may be contingently dependent upon human beings for survival, e.g., a dog or cat. However, dogs and cats can and, in fact, do survive and develop without human care. Only humans necessarily need the care of other humans to survive and develop. I discuss animal welfare issues in detail in 'Care Ethics and Animal Welfare' (2007).

'humanity' are beside the point, as are appeals to special characteristics. Logical consistency requires that we treat like cases the same, and since our own claims for caring stem from nothing other than our need for human care, we are logically committed to provide care to all other creatures who necessarily depend on human care for their survival, development, and functioning.

Gewirth's argument has also been criticized for reducing morality to logic, and a similar criticism might be leveled against my argument. E. J. Bond writes that 'Gewirth and others like him would turn wickedness into a kind of intellectual incompetence' (Bond 1980: 41). Gewirth seems to suggest that what is wrong with treating others immorally is not so much the harm we do them as the illogic or inconsistency of our actions. Deryck Beyleveld argues, however, that this criticism rests on a misunderstanding of Gewirth's argument: 'Irrationality (illogicality) is not what makes an action immoral [for Gewirth]. It is, however, the means by which we can know what actions are immoral' (Beyleveld 1991: 104). What makes an action immoral for Gewirth is that it deprives individuals of the freedom and well-being that all agents necessarily and universally depend upon to achieve their purposes. Logic merely provides a means for recognizing and explaining why certain actions are wrong. A similar sort of defense can be applied to the principle of consistent dependency. If we are to act consistently and nonhypocritically, all capable individuals should care for others in need. Yet, what is immoral about withholding care from others in need is not the inconsistency of our action but the fact that in doing so we deprive them of the support necessary for their survival, development, and functioning. We contribute to (if only by failing to prevent) the destruction or degradation of other people's lives, and implicitly renounce the basic practices and values that make our own lives, the reproduction of society, and the propagation of humanity (as we know it) possible, even though we all implicitly recognize these goals and practices as good. In short, what is immoral about refusing to care for others is that it involves us in acting contrary to moral principles that we are all implicitly committed to by the very nature of our dependent existence. The logic of the argument merely helps us to understand why actions that most people intuitively consider immoral (doing nothing when we could easily save a drowning child) are in fact so. They are contrary to the moral principles that necessarily follow from the dependent nature of human existence and are necessary to sustain human life.

The upshot of this argument is that all individuals have a right to care.[22] We can all make valid—that is, justifiable—claims on others for care when we need it.[23] Because we can morally validate our claims on others for care, we can all be said to have a right to care when we need it. Care theorists have generally been reluctant to use rights language in describing caring responsibilities on the grounds that rights discourse can be abstract, atomistic, and agonistic (Gilligan 1982; Hirschmann 1992; Noddings 1984; Robinson 1999). Yet, there are many different ways of conceiving of rights, and as the foregoing argument should make clear, rights language need not be framed in narrow individualistic terms. A conception of rights can be developed out of our dependency on others that promotes caring and relationships rather than separation and atomism (Hirschmann 2003: 158–69; Minow 1990: 227–372; Noddings 2002: 53–68).[24] The notion of a right to care is simply a shorthand way of indicating that individuals in need can justify their claims on others for care, and consequently, that capable individuals have an obligation to care for individuals in need when they can do so.

Thomas Hobbes famously suggested that human beings' desire for survival gives rise to a number of natural duties and rights. Care theorists have criticized Hobbes for failing to recognize the social dependency of human beings and the important role of caring in maintaining individual life and society (Held 1993: 195). Yet, if Hobbes had acknowledged human dependency and the important role of caring in maintaining individual life and society, he might have formulated an argument much like the preceding one. The value we place on our lives and functioning combined with our unavoidable dependency upon the care of others generates duties in us to care for others in need, and gives us the right to demand care from others when we need it. All capable individuals have a duty to help others meet their biological and developmental needs because we all depend upon the care of others for our survival, development, and functioning, and because denying others the care they need to survive,

---

[22] Robin West similarly discusses a 'right to care', but focuses on the right to give rather than receive care, and attempts to justify this right within a liberal, and specially American constitutional, framework (West 2002).

[23] For this idea of rights as justifiable or valid claims, see Feinberg (1970b).

[24] It is noteworthy that both Hirschmann and Noddings, who previously criticized rights discourse, now support its use for care theory. Hirschmann explains in a note that her earlier critique of rights 'was a critique of the classical liberal vision but did not preclude the feminist rethinking of rights' (2003: 268 n. 52). Her more recent work has focused on this issue.

develop, and function deprives them of the opportunity to attain goals that we all implicitly recognize as good.

## 1.3. The Distribution of Our Caring Duties

Section 1.1 of this chapter outlined a minimalist definition of caring that describes the core aims of a wide variety of commonly recognized caring practices and applies cross-culturally, and Section 1.2 developed a theory of obligation based upon this definition of caring. In ensuing chapters, I identify the institutions and policies that follow from this account of caring in the areas of domestic politics, economics, international relations, and culture. Before turning to these topics, however, one last subject remains to be addressed: the distribution of our caring duties. Given limitations of time, money, and other resources, we cannot care equally for everyone. We need guidelines for ordering our caring priorities since our caring obligations would otherwise be overwhelming (Held 1993: 74–5). Care theorists have noted this fact but have not very clearly outlined an account of the proper distribution of our caring duties.[25] In this final section, I develop a distributional framework for our caring duties based upon Robert Goodin's 'assigned responsibility' model of moral obligation, and further clarify a number of issues regarding the nature of our responsibilities to others (Goodin 1985: 109–44; 1995: 280–7).

Goodin begins his account of the assigned responsibility model with the assumption that we all have general moral duties to others. He then argues that many of our special moral duties are best understood as 'distributed general duties' (Goodin 1995: 280). Distributed general duties are general moral duties 'that, for one reason or another, are pursued more effectively if they are subdivided and particular people are assigned special responsibility for particular portions of the task' (Goodin 1995: 282). Goodin suggests, for example, that we all have a duty to protect the vulnerable. Yet, if everyone were to try to protect all vulnerable individuals equally, we would generally fulfill our duties less effectively than if we divided up these duties and assigned particular individuals special responsibility for protecting particular vulnerable persons. It is usually better to assign one doctor the particular care of each patient

---

[25] Friedman provides the best discussion of these issues (Friedman 1993: 9–88). My discussion mirrors hers in many respects, but provides a more precise account of our caring duties and builds upon my own account of caring.

in a hospital rather than assigning all doctors equal responsibility for all patients. If we were to assign all doctors the care of all patients, the likely result would be confusion, inefficiency, and less attentive care for all. In the *Politics*, Aristotle makes a similar point about the care of the young. 'People are more prone to neglect their duty when they think that another is attending to it.' If all adults were made equally responsible for the care of all children, 'the result will be that all will equally neglect them' (1995: 42, 1261b). Based upon these considerations, Goodin argues that our general duties to others in many cases dictate that we assign particular responsibilities to particular individuals as the best (or at least only practicable) means for fulfilling them. We are even justified under this scheme in showing some partiality toward our special dependents on the grounds that all dependents will generally be better protected if each protector shows some partiality toward his or her special dependents (e.g. taking special care to make sure they are fed or rescued from a burning building). An important correlate of this argument, however, is that we all have residual responsibilities for protecting other vulnerable individuals whose particular protectors fail to fulfill their duties toward them (Goodin 1985: 151–3, 1995: 282). The particular distribution of our general moral duties is merely a means for fulfilling these general duties and, as such, does not override them. We all become responsible once again for particular others when the particular persons assigned to look after them fail to perform their responsibilities.

Goodin uses his assigned responsibility model to explain our special duties to vulnerable individuals and fellow countrymen, but it applies equally well (if not better) to the distribution of our moral duties under care theory. As argued above, all capable individuals have duties to care for all individuals in need. Since, however, caring is best practiced in particular relationships where caregivers can be attentive, responsive, and respectful to those needing care, care theory favors a particular distribution of our caring duties. We can usually ensure the best care for all individuals by dividing up our general caring duties and assigning particular individuals primary responsibility for the care of particular others. Consistent with the assigned responsibility model, however, we still retain residual responsibilities to care for all others who may need our help. Our particular caring duties to particular others do not erase our general duties to all others, but represent only the best practical means for fulfilling them.

Drawing upon the assigned responsibility model, we may identify our primary responsibility under care theory as caring for ourselves. Capable individuals have a primary responsibility to care for themselves as much as possible because they are usually best able to determine and provide for their own particular needs—at least, that is, if they have adequate resources and opportunities to do so. They usually know better than others when they are hungry or cold and can usually best identify what will best nourish or warm them. Self-care also precedes and sustains caring for others. A person who does not care adequately for himself or herself may eventually be unable or unwilling to care for others. By caring for ourselves, we also avoid needlessly calling upon others to care for us, thereby allowing social resources to be directed toward the individuals who most need them.

This priority of self-care does not mean all acts of self-sacrifice are wrong. In certain well-defined cases where one must choose between the care of self and others, and one's own needs and the needs of the other party can be equally well met by the available resources or options, one might choose to sacrifice one's own care for the care of the other party. Because we can care equally well for ourselves or others in this case, the main justification for the priority of self-care over the care of others does not apply. Yet, these acts of self-sacrificing caring are always supererogatory since, as noted above, our obligations to care for others do not extend to actions that would endanger our own lives, compromise our long-term functioning, or undermine our ability to care for others.

Our secondary caring responsibilities are owed to individuals with whom we share some sort of special relationship or are in a special position to help. Most usually, this means our children, parents, spouses, partners, friends, and other intimate relations. We have special responsibilities to care for these individuals because we are usually best situated to provide them with the most attentive, responsive, and respectful care. We are also likely to have a relational history with them that may allow us to better understand and anticipate their needs and may make them more comfortable expressing their needs to us. Inasmuch as we feel affection for our intimate relations, we will also be motivated to provide them with more attentive, responsive, and respectful care than others are likely to provide. For all these reasons, we can usually most efficiently expend our resources (money, time, and energy) on caring for our family and friends. Our secondary duties may nonetheless also include individuals outside our family and friends depending upon circumstances. If we were to come across an injured hiker on a remote nature trail, we would have a special duty to care for this person, even though he or she might be a complete stranger, simply because of his or her circumstantial dependency upon us. Doctors, nurses, elder care workers, and other care workers are likewise specially responsible for the care of their patients or clients because they have agreed to attend to their needs.

After ourselves and individuals with whom we share a special relationship or are in a special position to help, we are next responsible for caring for individuals with whom we live in close proximity or share some sort of social relationship (community members and compatriots). Once again, we are most likely to know and understand the particular needs and capabilities of these individuals and are usually best positioned to care for them. Marilyn Friedman writes on this point:

There are, to be sure, some reasons on behalf of favoring the interests of neighbors and acquaintances, even those with resources, over the interests of unknown strangers. When one is acquainted with someone, then one knows something, however minimal, about her. One may be familiar with her needs, wants, situation, or the like. Knowing something about someone's particular circumstances makes it easier to help or care for her effectively than if one knows nothing in particular about her. In such cases of greater familiarity, the risk is lessened that the help or care one renders will be ineffective or, worse yet, detrimental to the recipient. (Friedman 1993: 57–8)

It may be added that our special responsibilities to ourselves and our family and friends also justify some partiality to those who live in our direct social environment. Individuals who live in our direct social environment are likely to become the partners, associates, friends, and caretakers of us and our loved ones. If we may be said to have a particular moral duty to care for ourselves and our intimate relations, then we must also have a particular moral duty to care for those in our immediate social environment, since caring for the latter will contribute to our own and our loved one's safety and care.

*care ethics = inherently selfish? individual-istic*

We finally have general duties to care for all others in need. These duties fall last in line because we are usually least well able and least well positioned to deliver good care to distant strangers. We may not understand the particular nature of these individuals' needs or may not be able very easily to provide the care they require. We may also have very little direct control over the social institutions and policies that determine the distribution of resources in distant countries. Consequently, our resources for caring are usually most efficiently expended closer to home. Nonetheless, we do have a duty to care for distant others when we are able to do so. The goal in caring for distant others should follow the pattern outlined above.

Because individuals are usually best able to care for themselves and those near them, we should aim to care for distant others whenever possible by enabling them to care for themselves and their immediate dependents as well as other individuals in their immediate social milieu. In this regard, care theory supports the principle of subsidiarity, or idea that we should shift the actual delivery of care whenever possible to the most local and personal levels. We should care for others whenever possible by enabling them to care for themselves.

The above framework describes in general terms the proper distribution of our caring obligations and more specifically explains why we might justifiably give priority to the care of ourselves, family, friends, and compatriots over others. It does not, however, provide an account of particular individuals' responsibilities to particular others. As Goodin notes, an additional 'responsibility principle' is necessary to indicate who in particular has a duty to care for whom: 'We cannot always deduce from considerations of general duties alone who in particular should take it on themselves to discharge them; where the general principle leaves that question open, some further (independent, often largely arbitrary) "responsibility principle" is required to specify it' (Goodin 1995: 280). Based upon the above framework, we can say that a person is justified in caring for a sick family member rather than using his or her resources to care for a sick distant stranger, but we cannot say without further information that one particular person (rather than, say, his or her brother or sister, or stepfather, or someone else) is primarily obligated to care for the ailing family member. Who in particular has a particular obligation to care for a specific person depends upon a number of largely circumstantial factors, including: the nature of their relationship; the proximity in which the potential caregiver lives to the person in need; whether others might also help the person in need; whether the potential caregiver has taken some self-assumed action that indicates to others that he or she intends to take responsibility for the dependent individual; social conventions and customary norms; and other factors.

While the specific nature of our obligations to particular others therefore remains indeterminate, care theory can offer several general guidelines for a responsibility principle. First, we assume a special obligation to do our best to provide at least adequate care for individuals when we take some action that indicates our intention to take on primary responsibility for their care. When individuals choose to raise a child—for example, by keeping a newborn baby rather than putting him or her up for adoption— then they assume special responsibility for the child's care. Since others are likely to assume that the child is being cared for by his or her parents, the child may die or suffer long-term disability if the parents fail to fulfill their self-assumed obligations. Alternatively, though, our special obligations to particular others should never force us to sacrifice our own health, safety, or functioning. Social conventions or customs that assign certain individuals the care of others are only morally justifiable insofar as they do not seriously undermine the caregiver's ability to meet his or her own needs (Friedman 1993: 44–52). Conventions that assign women primary responsibility for the care of children, elderly parents, and other dependent individuals and in the process make them vulnerable to abuse, poverty, and other harms are therefore invalid (Okin 1989a). Individuals have no moral obligation to abide by these conventions, though they may feel social pressure to do so. Finally, whatever the specific nature of our particular obligations to others, no individual should be expected to care for another inevitably dependent person wholly on his or her own. Under care theory, we all have obligations to provide support for individuals in need and their caregivers. Public subsidies and support services should be made available to all individuals in need to help them to fulfill their particular caring duties toward others and to ensure their adequate care.

The above framework describes the rightful distribution of our caring duties, but leaves a number of difficult questions unanswered. If we have only enough resources (time, money, and energy) to care for ourselves and our immediate dependents, then we are justified in devoting all our resources there. Similarly, if we have only enough resources to care for ourselves, our dependents, and our compatriots, then we are justified in caring only for them. Better to care for those individuals whose needs we can meet most effectively than to pass over needy individuals to care (usually less effectively) for distant others. Difficult questions arise, however, when we attempt to lend more specificity to these general principles. How much, for example, might individuals justifiably expend on the care of themselves and their dependents before turning to the care of others? Furthermore, are individuals justified in devoting some of their resources to toys for their children, symphony tickets, or religious pursuits even when distant others cannot meet their basic biological and developmental needs? Finally, what is our responsibility to individuals who are capable of caring for themselves but refuse to do so? The remainder of this chapter will address these questions.

The first question regarding morally justifiable expenditures on care for ourselves and our dependents raises a larger question about adequate threshold levels of caring. As noted above, there are certain objective levels of need satisfaction that set an absolute floor for caring. Individuals should at least have access to the basic goods and personal attention necessary to survive, develop, and function in society as much as possible without pain or suffering. What constitutes an adequate level of basic goods and personal attention, however, may vary somewhat according to social context and cultural norms. Different societies have different understandings of what exactly constitutes adequate food, clothing, housing, and other goods. The resources necessary for preparing individuals for social functioning may also vary somewhat depending on the nature of the society. In some societies, individuals may need a basic understanding of computers in order to function adequately in society, and in other societies, a basic understanding of farming or weaving techniques may be necessary. Different societies, then, may have reasonably different threshold levels of adequate caring based upon what is necessary to survive, develop, and function in their social context. Individuals are morally justified at least in expending a level of resources on themselves and others sufficient to meet this threshold of adequate care. In practice, this means that individuals in one society might justifiably spend much more on the care of themselves and others than individuals in another society. While individuals in wealthy societies should also take steps to improve the opportunities for individuals in poorer societies, especially when it would foster better caring for poor individuals, they need not do so at the cost of providing less than adequate care for themselves and others in their home societies. An individual who cannot achieve basic functioning in one society is not necessarily any better off than an individual who cannot reach this goal in another society even though their circumstances may be very different.

The second question raised above asks whether individuals are justified in devoting some resources above a socially-defined threshold of adequate care to purchase toys for their children, attend the symphony, support their religion, or most generally pursue their ideal of the good life.[26] Peter Singer argues on utilitarian grounds that individuals and societies have an obligation to devote all resources above those necessary for their basic well-being to the subsistence needs of distant others (Singer 1993:

---

[26] As noted above, some expenditures on sports, art, piano lessons and the like might be justified on the grounds that they are necessary to help children or others to develop or maintain their basic capabilities for emotion, affiliation, imagination, and so forth. I am focusing here on additional expenditures that aim to develop complex capabilities or foster some idea of the good.

218–46). By his account, we act immorally when we spend $200 to attend the symphony or eat dinner at an expensive restaurant rather than using this money to save the life of a starving child abroad. On the face of it, care theory might seem to endorse a similar principle. Since we have a moral obligation to care for all others in need, it might seem wrong to spend our resources on any conception of the good life when there are literally billions of people around the world who can barely survive. Even taking into account the inefficiencies and hazards of caring for distant others, it would seem morally obligatory at least to try to help others to meet their basic survival and developmental needs before expending any resources on toys, symphony tickets, or religious pursuits.[27]

While this position may follow from Singer's account of utilitarianism, it is not supported by the account of care theory outlined above. If care theory were to require that individuals devote themselves wholly to the care of all individuals before devoting any resources to other goods, then it would come to resemble an all-encompassing conception of the good life, subordinating all other moral ideals to its goals. We would all be obligated to devote virtually all of our resources to the care of others and none to play, aesthetic appreciation, religious pursuits, or other goods, since we can almost always do more to care for others. There is, however, nothing in the nature of care theory to justify this sort of moral predominance. The practice of caring is prior to and necessary for any conception of the good life, and as such, serves as a sort of internal check on all conceptions of morality and the good life. Any moral theory or conception of the good life that denies the importance of caring practices or directly subverts them may be said to be internally inconsistent and immoral. But this does not mean that caring duties should assume predominance over all other values. There are many legitimate values and ends of human life other than those associated with caring, and caring values cannot be shown to be always more important than all other pursuits. Some people might consider tithing to their church more important than contributing funds to feed the hungry, and others might feel the same about toys for their children and symphony tickets for themselves. Since caring for others cannot be shown to be always more important than these other aims, we cannot be said to be morally obligated to provide adequate care to all individuals before devoting any resources to developing the higher capabilities of our loved ones or pursuing some conception of the good

---

[27] I further discuss some of the hazards of foreign aid and how they relate to a caring foreign policy in Chapter 4.

life. Yet, we do have general duties to care for all others in need regardless of our vision of the good life, and the more resources we devote to our vision of the good life or developing the complex capabilities of ourselves or our children, the fewer resources we will have available to devote to the care of others. At the very least, then, if we have sufficient resources to support one form of a good life or another, we should also devote some resources to caring for others. Care theory does not place the duty to care for others above all other visions of the good life, but it does identify caring as a basic moral duty that all individuals and peoples should at least balance against their other goals and values. [28]

BALANCE.

While this idea of balancing our moral duties of caring with conceptions of the good life might seem strange, it is actually in line with generally accepted moral practices. Nearly all people and societies consider murder to be wrong, for example, and recognize a general obligation to devote some resources to protect against it. Yet, no one suggests that we ought to devote all our resources to guarding painstakingly against murder. We balance the very important moral duty to prevent murder with other goods. So it is with caring. Caring for others is a fundamental moral duty that deserves our constant attention and some portion of our disposable resources. But caring cannot be shown conclusively to be the only activity worth doing. It is a basic duty but not necessarily the overriding good of human existence. We thus must balance our duties to care with other ideas of the good life.

This notion of balancing our duty to care with other visions of the good life confronts at least one fundamental objection. If individuals can legitimately devote some of their resources to their pursuit of the good life before donating to the care of others, then it might seem justifiable for parents to devote some resources to pursuing their conception of the good life even at the cost of providing adequate care for their children. This conclusion does not follow from the argument above, however, because of the responsibility principle outlined earlier. When we take some action that indicates our intention to take on primary responsibility for the care of individuals, we assume a special obligation to do our best to provide at least adequate care for them. Part of assuming primary responsibility for a dependent individual involves a willingness to put aside one's pursuit of the good life when necessary to ensure the dependent individual's minimally adequate care. Individuals who choose to raise a child thus

---

[28] Slote argues that we must balance our self-concern, our care of loved ones, and our care for others (2001: 69–78). Here I extend this idea to argue that we must also balance our caring obligations with our conceptions of the good.

assume special responsibility for the child's care, including the responsibility to ensure his or her adequate care before devoting any resources to the pursuit of the good life. Adequate care trumps the pursuit of the good life in intimate, self-assumed relations because of the special obligations involved.

We finally must consider our duties to individuals who, although fully capable, make no efforts to care for themselves (Kymlicka 1990: 277–84). As noted above, I depart from Kari Waerness in distinguishing personal services from necessary caring (Waerness 1984). In my account, a person who helps others to meet their basic needs, develop or sustain their basic capabilities, or alleviate their pain or suffering cares for them whether the cared-for could have fulfilled these needs by himself or herself. However, in the general spirit of Waerness's distinction, I agree that personal service-type care is not obligatory. That is, while it might be caring of us to make dinner for a perfectly capable spouse or friend, we are under no moral obligation to do so. The reasoning for this position follows from the argument outlined above. Our legitimate rights claims for caring are based upon our generic dependency on others for care. Since all people can be assumed to have claimed care from others only when it was necessary for their survival, development, and basic functioning, we can validate our own claims for care only when we really need it for our survival, development, and basic functioning. Individuals who call upon us to care for them when they are not really in need ('Make me dinner!', 'Get me some water!') thus cannot validate their right claim. Our care for them, if we so choose to care for them, is strictly beneficent.

Since our duty to care for others arises only in cases of need, some further clarification is necessary for describing what exactly constitutes need. The criterion for distinguishing real needs is certainly not whether we would need care in a particular situation (e.g. 'As a former Olympic swimmer I would not need to be saved from drowning in such calm waters'). Rather, the criterion is whether it would be difficult for a particular individual in a particular situation to achieve an important caring aim (food, water, safety, and the development of basic capabilities) without our help. If it seems unlikely that the person could achieve a caring aim without our help, then we should offer care to him or her.[29] This applies importantly even to individuals who need our care because of unwise choices they may have made in the past. Robert Goodin writes in this regard:

---

[29] These points are further discussed in Chapter 2.

The notion of desert is ordinarily...out of place in deciding how to judge the improvident. They should be regarded as foolhardy people whose recklessness is to be discouraged through appropriate disincentives, not as evil people whose wickedness deserves to be punished. When dealing with people in precarious situations, questions of fault are simply out of place. (Goodin 1985: 133)

If an ice skater recklessly skates on to thin ice and falls into the water, he or she still deserves to be saved. Similarly, if individuals find themselves at some point in their lives incapable of caring for themselves because of poor educational or business choices, they still deserve our care—in this case, probably in the form of temporary assistance and job training. There are nonetheless some reasonable limits on whom we are obligated to care for. Care theory does not justify, for example, a basic minimum income for capable individuals who refuse to work or care for others (Van Parijs 1998). This limitation on our duty to care is important because it protects caregivers against the potential exploitation that always exists in caring relationships and can undermine people's willingness to care even for individuals who truly need our help. As argued in Chapter 2, there are nonetheless some practical policy reasons for offering at least some basic caring services to all individuals without attaching complicated eligibility requirements to them. From a strictly moral perspective, however, we have no duty to care for capable individuals who refuse to make reasonable efforts to care for themselves.

## 1.4. Conclusion

In this chapter, I have tried to clarify and sharpen our understanding of care theory by specifying what it means to care and explaining why and for whom we have duties to care. Caring means most basically helping individuals to meet their basic needs, develop or sustain their basic capabilities, and avoid and alleviate unwanted suffering in attentive, responsive, and respectful ways. The ultimate aim is to enable individuals to survive and function in society so that they can care for themselves and others and pursue some conception of the good life.

While my account of caring might appear quite different from Gilligan's and Noddings's original definitions, it still shares some important elements with them. Gilligan argued, for example, that caring involves a sense of responsibility for others and desire to alleviate the 'real and recognizable trouble' of the world (Gilligan 1982: 30, 100). Noddings associated her original account of caring with meeting the basic needs of others

(Noddings 1984). The definition of caring outlined here simply specifies in a more precise way the sorts of needs that a caring person addresses. My account of caring also preserves the element of contextual reasoning that is so important to Gilligan's and Noddings's original definitions. Caring, as I have defined it, means meeting vital needs, fostering basic capabilities, and alleviating suffering with close attention to context and differences among individuals, that is, in attentive, responsive, and respectful ways.

All capable individuals have a duty to care for others in need because we are all dependent upon others for care and at least implicitly have made claims on others for care. Indeed, our desire for survival and functioning along with our inevitable dependency makes caring for others in need a moral goal written into the very fabric of our existence. Our primary caring duties are owed to ourselves and individuals who are close to us emotionally and geographically, but we also have residual duties to care for all other individuals in need of care.

The next step in the argument is to identify the social institutions and policies that follow from this account of caring. I begin to address these issues in Chapter 2 by describing the political institutions and policies that support personal and social caring. Even where political institutions and policies do not support caring, however, we all have a personal duty to care for others in need when we are able to do so. Caring for others is a minimal basic morality that we owe to all individuals by virtue of our common human nature as dependent social creatures.

relatable to Camus?
can't kill others b/c
we value life

must care for others b/c
we expect care

65

# 2

# Care Theory and Domestic Politics

Early care theorists resisted applying care ethics to politics on the grounds that any effort to manifest the commitments of caring in general institutions and policies would invariably distort its nature. More recent care theorists, however, have noted important flaws in this approach to caring (see Introduction), and identified a number of ways in which political institutions and policies can manifest caring values. Specifically, political institutions and policies can establish the background conditions necessary for personal caring, lend support to personal caring practices, and, if properly organized, provide care to individuals in need. Yet, despite the important groundwork that has been done in preparing the way for a political theory of caring, a general account of the basic institutions and policies of a caring society remains underdeveloped.

Among care theorists, Joan Tronto has been one of the most important proponents of the idea that care ethics can and should inform political theory (Fisher and Tronto 1990; Tronto 1987, 1993, 1996, 1998). In *Moral Boundaries* and a number of articles, she identified a number of problems with the early definitions of caring, outlined an influential definition of the practice of caring, and demonstrated that care can be connected to a theory of justice and used to guide policymaking. As noted in Chapter 1, however, her definition of caring is too broad to provide clear guidance on moral and political issues. Her political theory of care is also vague.

Tronto argues most generally that 'care is only viable as a political ideal in the context of liberal, pluralistic, democratic institutions' because care presupposes 'a politics in which there is, at the center, a public discussion of needs, and an honest appraisal of the intersection of needs and interests' (Tronto 1993: 158, 168). Institutional principles such as the rule of law, the protection of rights, and due process 'constitute a part of care' because they promote 'listening and responding' and allow citizens to articulate and discuss their needs (Tronto 1993: 215, n. 6). Yet, as Tronto readily admits, liberal democratic institutions are not sufficient for achieving a caring polity. If they were, there would be no need for care theory to supplement them. Tronto therefore further stipulates that a caring political theory is one where 'care as a practice can inform the practices of democratic citizenship' (1993: 167). Caring democratic citizens will be concerned with 'employment policies, nondiscrimination, equalizing expenditures in schools, providing adequate access to health care' and generally making sure 'that all people are adequately cared for' (Tronto 1996: 145). Unfortunately, Tronto does not elaborate upon these ideas in any detail, and ultimately provides only the barest sketch of what a caring polity might look like.

In her recent work *Starting at Home: Caring and Social Policy* (2002), Noddings has revised her earlier position on caring to argue that care ethics can in fact guide social policymaking (1). She still insists on the supreme moral value of personal caring, but now adds that institutional forms of caring, or caring-about, are also important (22). In particular, she argues that political institutions and policies should be 'seen as instrumental in establishing the conditions under which caring-for can flourish' (23). By supporting institutions and policies that lend support to personal caring, we can care 'for others by working to establish social conditions in which care can flourish' (48).

Noddings begins her discussion of political institutions and policies by 'starting at home' and examining the types of caring practices that are found in the best home environments (1). The most caring homes attend to the needs of dependents, foster their growth, train them for social acceptance, and avoid causing pain or using coercion whenever possible. Based upon these aims, Noddings formulates a number of policy proposals for developing a more caring society. Her first priority is finding homes for the homeless, since homes are central to meeting many of our basic needs including shelter, safety, food, and medical care (249–51). She argues that governments should support the construction of apartment or dorm complexes for homeless individuals, the creation of permanent group homes for the mentally ill, and emergency loans for individuals in danger of losing their homes (248–64). Noddings also calls for the reform of the school curriculum to include classes designed to teach students about parenting, child development, nutrition, and other household skills (283–300).[1] She adds that both abortion and euthanasia should be legal,

---

[1] Noddings's educational philosophy is further discussed in Chapter 5.

but subject to certain restrictions and mandatory counseling (235–9). Conversely, the war on drugs and capital punishment should be abolished since both are excessively punitive and cruel (243–7, 269–78). These recommendations form the central pillars of Noddings's political theory. Since her aim is to show how an ethic of care might be infused into existing liberal societies, she can hardly be faulted for her partial and somewhat idiosyncratic discussion of topics (229–30). Yet her argument falls short of developing a full account of the basic political institutions of a caring society.

Eva Kittay offers a somewhat different approach to developing a caring political theory. She suggests that a caring social policy should be organized around the principle of *doulia*, a term taken from the name of the postpartum caregiver (a doula) who assists the new mother as the mother cares for the infant (Kittay 1999: 68). She defines the principle of *doulia* as follows: 'Just as we have required care to survive and thrive, so we need to provide conditions that allow others—including those who do the work of caring—to receive the care they need to survive and thrive' (107). In terms of social policy, she recommends establishing social institutions and programs that provide aid and support to caregivers and their dependents much as a doula might do for a new mother (108). She praises, for example, the US Family and Medical Leave Act (FMLA) of 1993, which permits up to twelve weeks of unpaid leave for workers within any twelve month period in order to care for a new child or sick or disabled family member. Yet she argues that this policy is marred by three shortcomings: '1) leave is unpaid; 2) employers with less than 50 employees are exempt from the FMLA; 3) the FMLA construes family in relatively traditional terms' (135). Because of these shortcomings, the majority of the workforce is unable to take advantage of this law. An immediate solution would be to provide monetary subsidies for workers during their leave time, expand the FMLA to include all employees, and allow nonmarried adults who are cohabitating to qualify for it. More radically, Kittay calls for a 'socialization and a universalization of compensation for dependency work' in the form of a public subsidy for care work 'which can be used to compensate a mother for her time caring for her child, or allow her to use the money to pay for day care. Or to provide a son or daughter to care for an ailing parent, or to pay someone else to perform the service' (143). While this policy—or something like it—surely represents an important element of a caring political theory, it is only one part of it. Like other care theorists, Kittay does not discuss the larger institutional context of a caring government.

Other care theorists have similarly defended a variety of social policies designed to support caring practices (Cancian and Oliker 2000; Clement 1996; Fineman 2004; Folbre 2001; Harrington 1999; Held 1993; Kittay and Feder 2002; Robinson 1999; Ruddick 1989; Sevenhuijsen 1998; West 1997; White 2000).[2] Like Kittay, however, most theorists discuss only a few particular policies usually in relation to one specific country or another. Few theorists have examined the basic political institutions of a caring society. Consequently, the political theory of caring remains something less than a full theory of justice.

This chapter takes up the task of describing the basic political institutions and policies of a caring society. I examine how the aims and virtues of caring can be embodied in the political framework of society, and how political institutions and policies can be used to provide care to individuals and support personal caring practices. I begin by addressing a question that care theorists have not satisfactorily answered: why should government assume responsibility for supporting caring activities at all? As argued in Chapter 1, we all have a moral duty to care for others; but insofar as we can fulfill this duty outside of the government institutions, there would seem to be no justification for a political theory of caring. The first part of this chapter explains why we should shift at least some of our caring duties to the government. I then describe the central principles of a caring government, and outline in some detail the specific institutions and policies necessary for providing individuals with at least minimally adequate care. Since any discussion of minimally adequate care will inevitably raise questions about cultural bias, I next discuss the relation between care theory and multiculturalism. In Section 2.6, I address a number of possible objections to the implementation of a caring government, including concerns about its costs and the potential for abuse in some caring programs.

## 2.1. Caring as a Political Value

Caring, as defined in Chapter 1, involves everything we do directly to help individuals to meet their basic needs, develop or sustain their basic capabilities, and minimize or alleviate unwanted suffering. Basic needs include food, sanitary water, clothing, shelter, rest, a clean environment, basic medical care, and protection from harm, as well as the need at

[2] This chapter focuses on domestic political justice. Economic issues (Folbre and Held) and international relations (Robinson and Ruddick) are discussed in Chapters 3 and 4.

least among infants for physical contact and affection. Basic capabilities include the ability to sense, move about, feel, imagine, reason, communicate, affiliate with others, and in most societies, read, write, and perform basic math. We all have a duty to care for others because we are all dependent upon the care of others for our survival, development, and basic social functioning. Since we have all made claims on others for care and continue to do so, it is inconsistent and immoral by our own implicit moral standards to ignore or deny the claims of others for care when we can help them.

Although we have a moral duty to care for others in need, this does not necessarily mean that we ought to make caring a part of the political structure of society. Most of us recognize a variety of moral duties such as the duty to tell the truth or to be faithful to our spouses or partners that we generally do not look to government to enforce. In fact, the duty to care has long been considered a private or personal moral duty that rightfully falls outside the scope of governmental jurisdiction. Why then should we involve the government in caring?

Robert Goodin's discussion of collective responsibilities is useful in answering this question (1985: 134–44). In *Protecting the Vulnerable*, he argues that we have moral duties to protect all individuals who are vulnerable to our actions. In many cases, we can best fulfill our responsibilities by individually looking after others, but in other cases we can only or most competently fulfill our responsibilities through collective organizations. Individuals who live near a coast where boats regularly capsize, for example, may be said to have a responsibility to save drowning boaters (136–7). Assuming, however, that no individual can save the drowning boaters by himself or herself, Goodin argues that these individuals have a responsibility to organize a collective rescue scheme, such as establishing and maintaining a lifeboat and crew. While the usual excuses for not helping others such as 'there's nothing I can do by myself' may absolve individuals of individual responsibility, they usually succeed only by pointing to a more general group obligation (Goodin 1989: 126). If it is right to do something that individuals cannot do alone but can accomplish through collective efforts, then individuals have a duty to organize collective efforts to do the right thing. Goodin concludes that individuals have a responsibility to organize and implement a collective scheme for protecting the vulnerable whenever their individual duties can only or best be fulfilled through collective schemes.

A similar argument can be applied to care theory. As argued in Chapter 1, we have general duties to care for all others in need when we are

71

capable of doing so. Our primary duties are owed to ourselves and those closest to us emotionally and spatially since we can usually care most attentively, responsively, and respectfully for these individuals. Yet we also have duties to care for others in our communities, society, and the world at large when we have the resources to do so. While we might attempt to care personally for these individuals, we cannot in many cases do so very effectively. It may be difficult to learn about the needs of individuals who live far away from us or to deliver goods or services to them. Many times, too, a person's needs may exceed the capabilities of any one caregiver. Many homeless individuals, for example, have a multitude of needs—for shelter, clothes, food, medical care, job training, etc.—that few individuals are capable of meeting on their own. As in the lifeboat example, the only way to care effectively for these individuals is by pooling resources and establishing collective caring organizations. Collective caring organizations can also more effectively gather information about distant others and deliver goods and services to them. Following Goodin, we thus may say that individuals have a duty to organize and support collective caring schemes when they can only or most effectively care for others through organized collective efforts. In many cases, these collective caring organizations will be the only means for fulfilling our moral obligation to care for others in need.

*can't do it alone*

The duty to organize collective schemes of care still does not commit us to institutionalizing caring in the basic political institutions of society. Individuals might, for example, organize and contribute to private or charitable schemes of collective care without resorting to government help. Such private or charitable organizations are fully consistent with the values of caring—at least insofar as they provide for the basic and developmental needs of individuals in attentive, responsive, and respectful ways. Nonetheless, there are several reasons for further institutionalizing collective care in the political structure of society.

First, there are some basic needs that only government, or a government-like entity, can effectively satisfy, including needs for safety and security, a clean environment, and other public goods. It seems unlikely that individuals could effectively fulfill their need for safety and security exclusively by hiring private security agencies to protect them. The overlapping jurisdictions and different rules of competing private security services would generate a great deal of uncertainty and conflict among people (Nozick 1974). Some individuals might also remain unprotected by this system. The only way effectively to ensure our own protection and the protection of others (whom we are responsible for looking after under care theory) is by supporting and complying with a government entity that possesses the authority to maintain peace and security for everyone within a territorial area.

A similar point can be made about environmental protections. As economists have long noted, individuals and private organizations are usually not very effective at securing public goods on their own because public goods by definition provide benefits to many individuals regardless of a person's efforts to achieve them. Many individuals may benefit from one individual's conscientious environmental practices, but the environmentally conscientious individual will bear all the costs and burdens. Most individuals may further find it cheaper and easier in the short term to engage in harmful and destructive environmental practices, especially if the costs of their actions can be shifted over to others. Some authoritative collective organizations are thus necessary to establish and enforce environmental regulations. Without government coordination and enforcement, it seems very unlikely that individuals could assure themselves and others of a clean and safe environment.

A second reason for institutionalizing at least some collective care activities in government is to ensure that the basic needs of all individuals are effectively met throughout society (Goodin 1985: 137–8).[3] While private organizations may help us to care adequately for some individuals, they are likely to result in the neglect of others unless coordinated by some central body. All of the bystanders on a crowded beach may have a duty to rescue a drowning swimmer, for example, but without some sort of coordination, 'the results would be confusing and chaotic, with hordes of rescuers getting in each other's way' (Feinberg 1970a: 244). The situation is far more complicated when applied to the care of all individuals within society. Numerous private care organizations may rise up in one locale but none in another; too many organizations may focus on homelessness and not enough on caring for people with disabilities. Government need not supplant the efforts of these private care organizations, but it can supplement and coordinate them by directing resources to underserved areas or setting up new programs in neglected areas to ensure that the needs of all individuals are satisfied. In this way, government can help us

---

[3] Goodin notes that the coordination problem does not necessarily require that government oversee the distribution of resources (1988: 155). A supersized charity could equally well collect contributions and distribute them as needed. However, when combined with the other considerations listed below—government's role in monitoring care and ensuring that everyone contributes their fair share to it—then government appears solely capable of effectively coordinating caring activities as well.

to fulfill our caring responsibilities to individuals who might otherwise be neglected.

The government can also help us to fulfill our caring responsibilities by monitoring care and providing residual care as necessary. As argued in Chapter 1, although we all have primary responsibilities to care for our close relations and friends, we nonetheless retain residual responsibilities to care for individuals whose appointed caregivers fail them or who have no primary caregiver. Along with this responsibility comes the duty to monitor, or remain attentive to, the well-being of other individuals to see if they need our care (Goodin 1985: 134–5). Few individuals, however, have the resources or authority to monitor and detect cases of abuse or neglect, or to intervene and (forcibly if necessary) take over the care of abused or neglected individuals. Only government usually has the requisite authority and resources to carry out these tasks. Our residual duty to care for others thus obligates us to set up a government body to identify and address situations where individuals are not receiving adequate care.

A final reason to institutionalize collective care in the political structure of society is to ensure that everyone contributes his or her fair share to it. While everyone has a moral duty to care for others according to his or her abilities, not everyone may voluntarily fulfill their moral obligations. If some individuals do not contribute their fair share to the care of others, in turn, individuals in need will receive lesser quality care or perhaps no care at all. Our duty to care for others thus includes a duty to compel other capable individuals to do their fair share to care for others in need. The best means to fulfill this aspect of our duty to care is through government. The government can establish general standards of fairness designating how much individuals should be expected to contribute to the care of others (tax rates) and can use the threat of force if necessary to compel compliance with these standards.[4] A purely private approach to caring, by contrast, would allow some immoral or misguided individuals to avoid contributing their fair share to the care of needy individuals, thereby diminishing the quality and quantity of caring for many people throughout society.

As the foregoing argument should make clear, a caring government will not attempt to take over the direct care of all individuals, but instead aim to supplement, support, and accommodate the caring activities and organizations that already exist throughout society. The central justification for its actions derives from our moral duty to care for others. In

---

[4] A system of just taxation under care theory is outlined in Chapter 3.

many cases, we can only or most competently fulfill our caring duties by supporting government institutions that can support personal caregiving activities and provide care to individuals in need. This principle of governmental responsibility for caring is really just the flip side of the principle of personal responsibility for caring as discussed in Chapter 1. Just as we have special duties to care for those who are closest to us because we can usually best care for them, so also we have a duty to delegate responsibility for at least some forms of caring to the government because in many cases we can only and most competently fulfill our duties to others (both near and far) through public institutions and policies. In care theory, government functions primarily as a collective moral entity that facilitates and extends our ability to care for ourselves and others.

## 2.2. The Principles of a Caring Government

Caring for others through political institutions, or collective caring, is obviously different from personal caring. Personal caring involves helping others to satisfy their biological and developmental needs in a face-to-face manner. Collective caring involves supporting institutions and policies that sustain personal caring relationships or provide personal care to individuals in need. The distinction here is similar to the one that Noddings draws between caring-for and caring-about. Whereas caring-for occurs in the 'face-to-face occasions in which one person, as carer, cares directly for another, the cared-for,' caring-about 'moves us from the face-to-face world into the wider public realm' where institutions and policies serve to establish and promote 'the conditions under which caring-for can flourish' (2002: 22–3). In collective or political caring, our contributions are smaller and more diffuse, but still count as caring insofar as they directly help others to meet their biological and developmental needs in attentive, responsive, and respectful ways. Although in collective caring we delegate the actual task of caring to agencies and social service workers, this seems not so very different from caring for a sick relation by hiring a doctor or nurse to look after him or her. We care for individuals in these cases by supporting good caregiving, rather than attempting to provide an inferior form of care ourselves. We do the same on a social level when we support and comply with collective caring institutions.

The aims of a caring government are the same as those of a caring person:

75

(1) To help individuals to meet their basic needs for nourishment, sanitary water, clothes, shelter, basic medical care, a clean environment, rest, and protection from physical harm when they cannot reasonably meet these needs on their own.

(2) To help individuals to develop and sustain their basic capabilities for sensation, mobility, emotion, imagination, reason, communication, affiliation, literacy, and numeracy when they cannot reasonably achieve these goals on their own.

(3) To help individuals to avoid and alleviate unnecessary pain and suffering when they need help in meeting this goal.

The overarching goal of a caring government, like a caring individual, is to help people survive, develop, and avoid unwanted or unnecessary pain or suffering so that they can function as much as possible in society, meaning that they can work, care for themselves and others, and pursue some conception of the good life.

A central question for a caring political theory is how to judge whether a person is in need or, alternatively, could reasonably meet his or her needs through his or her own efforts. As noted in Chapter 1, we cannot simply reflect upon our own abilities and opportunities to arrive at a general definition of need, since different individuals have different abilities and opportunities as well as different levels of need. Rather, we must focus on the particular individual and situation and ask whether he or she is likely to be able to achieve an important caring aim (food, water, or education) without the help of others or ourselves. In any given situation, there may be some room for debate about the sort of effort we might reasonably expect people to make in attempting to satisfy their needs. Some general guidelines can nonetheless be outlined. First, there are some basic needs that no individuals can reasonably satisfy on their own, such as the need for protection and a clean environment. Since it would at least be extremely difficult, if not impossible, for an individual to secure these goods without the cooperation of others, individuals can generally be said to need the help of others in obtaining them. Secondly, there are some states of being, such as childhood, disability, sickness, and frail old age, when no individuals can reasonably be expected to meet their needs on their own. Individuals' physical or mental incapacity during these periods—and in the case of medical care, the limited knowledge most individuals have about treating sickness—means they must rely on others to survive, develop, and function. Thirdly, most individuals who care for a child, disabled individual, or other inevitably dependent person depend in some way upon others to help them satisfy their needs. It would be extremely burdensome in most cases for an individual to provide adequate full-time intensive care to a dependent individual while also working to obtain the resources necessary to support this caring (and also finding adequate time to care for himself or herself). Finally, all human beings are subject to bad luck, reversals of fortune, and bad decisions that may leave us at least temporarily without adequate means or opportunities for meeting our needs. If individuals lack the means and opportunities for meeting their needs, they cannot reasonably be expected to meet their needs on their own. We should all be able to recognize as legitimate the needs that arise from one or more of these conditions, since few (if any) of us could satisfy our needs without the care of others in these situations. Other more particular considerations might further be relevant for assessing the need of individuals in specific cases, but these general considerations at least provide a general framework for thinking about what we might reasonably expect of others and ourselves.

A second important issue for a political theory of caring is how to determine standards of adequate care. Since the overarching aim of a caring government is to help people to achieve and maintain social functioning, governments should define standards of adequate care at levels adequate to meet this goal. In different societies, individuals may need different types and levels of goods and services to achieve and maintain functioning. Standards of adequate care may thus vary somewhat from society to society depending upon circumstances. In general, though, the standard of adequate care in any society should reflect the threshold of goods and services necessary to support the survival, development, and functioning of all individuals in their social context.

Because caring is usually only effective when individuals are attentive, responsive, and respectful toward others in need, a caring government must further find ways to incorporate these virtues into its policies. There are two main ways of doing so. First, a caring government should attempt whenever possible to involve the potential recipients of care in the process of formulating and implementing the policies designed to serve them. In addition to the three aims listed above, a fourth principle of a caring political theory may thus be stated as follows:

(4) When governments organize or fund programs to care directly for individuals or support caring relationships, they should aim to involve the potential care recipients as much as possible in formulating and running these programs. In this way, they can better

SOLUTION

ensure that the programs will be tailored to recipients' actual needs and utilize their talents. (White 2000)

There are a number of ways that governments might involve potential care recipients in program design and administration. At the very least, they should hold public hearings in order to allow potential care recipients to express their needs and make suggestions about how programs should be designed. Even better, governments might adopt community-organizing models for designing and implementing programs. Public officials might work with community members to identify needs within their community and then serve as liaisons between government agencies and the community members to establish local programs tailored to individuals' specific needs. Governments might also provide grants to already existing community organizations so that they can care for individuals within their communities in context-sensitive ways, or allow local administrators some leeway in adapting general programs to local concerns.

A second important strategy for incorporating the virtues of caring into government programs is encompassed by the principle of subsidiarity:

> (5) Governments should shift the delivery of care as much as possible to the personal and local level, facilitating the care of individuals primarily by providing support for parents, families, caregivers, and local organizations who can care for individuals in context-specific and particular ways.

As Kittay argues, governments should not attempt to function like the heads of a family, directly caring for all people under their jurisdiction (1999). Rather, they should function as much as possible like doulas, facilitating the ability of caregivers, families, and community organizations to provide particular care for individuals close to them. In this way, they can usually foster the most attentive, responsive, and respectful forms of care for individuals. In shifting caring to personal and local levels, governments nonetheless should not abdicate all responsibility over it. They are still responsible for monitoring caregiving and providing residual care to individuals who might need support (perhaps because local organizations or personal caregivers fail to meet their needs). Some forms of care, too, cannot be effectively decentralized (e.g. national defense and environmental protections). Whenever feasible, though, governments should aim to support personal and local caring rather than provide care directly itself, and design programs so that individuals have some choice in determining how to care for themselves and others.

The principle of subsidiarity under care theory should not be confused with conservative proposals to privatize caring (Murray 1984). While many conservatives argue that caring should be performed as much as possible by family, friends, and local organizations, they usually look to these groups not only to care for individuals but also to sustain the costs of care work by themselves. A caring government, by contrast, subsidizes personal, family, and local caring so that adequate care is more accessible to all, and spreads the costs of this support evenly across society. It favors personal and local caring, in other words, but still regards support for caring as a public responsibility.

The final principle of a caring government is the principle of public outreach. Within traditional welfare states, many individuals who are entitled to public benefits are either unaware of them or do not know how to access them (Goodin 1988: 215–17; White and Tronto 2004). In some cases, public officials have even been known to instruct government workers not to tell welfare recipients about some of the benefits available to them (Barry 2005: 160). These practices are obviously contrary to the aims and virtues of caring. The central aim of caring is to meet the biological and developmental needs of people. One of the central virtues of caring—attentiveness—further directs us to seek out and address needs that individuals may have but fail to verbalize or even fully recognize. Since poor and needy individuals are often in the worst position to access government services, caring governments should reach out to them and make it as easy as possible for them to access the resources they need. The sixth and final principle of a caring government can thus be stated as follows:

(6) Government should endeavor to make everyone aware of the programs that exist to support and accommodate caring, and should make access to these programs as easy as possible for all eligible individuals.

The best means for informing people about programs and ensuring easy access to them will vary quite a bit from one society to another. One general means, though, of making programs known and easily accessible is to make them universally open to all individuals.

## 2.3. The Basic Institutions of a Caring Government

The six principles listed above provide a general sense of the nature of a caring government, but do not provide a very concrete picture of its institutions and policies. In this section, I fill out the picture of a caring government by identifying its main substantive institutions and policies. I assume here the social background of an industrialized Western society, and concentrate at several points specifically on the United States. Care theory is certainly not limited to Western societies, and in fact many of the institutions and policies discussed below could be applied to almost any country. Some of the specific institutional and policy recommendations nonetheless would likely be different in non-Western and less developed countries.

The most general task of a caring government is to help individuals to satisfy their needs for a number of public goods that they cannot reasonably obtain on their own. A caring government will provide people with military and police protections, a clean and safe environment, sanitary water and sewage, basic infrastructure goods such as roads and bridges, and other public goods necessary to support healthy, productive, and caring lives. By providing these public goods, governments can help individuals to satisfy a number of their biological needs and further establish the social background conditions necessary for personal caring.

Consistent with this first general goal, a caring government will also guarantee all individuals a number of basic rights essential for their physical integrity and security. These rights include protections against unwarranted military or police violence, cruel and unusual punishment, torture, and arbitrary arrest and detention, as well as the right to a fair trial. These basic protections follow from the nature of caring itself. Caring involves helping individuals to survive, develop, function, and avoid suffering and pain whenever possible. A caring person or government will thus do nothing unnecessarily to harm individuals or deprive them of the opportunity to live and interact with others. While a caring government may legitimately detain and punish individuals who break the law, the reasons for doing so should be evident to all members in society. If individuals are subject to arbitrary government actions, their ability to care for themselves and their loved ones may be seriously compromised. Beatings, torture, and the like are also all self-evidently uncaring. A caring government will therefore ban these measures and take steps to protect individuals from possible abuses by its own officials.[5]

A caring government will similarly guarantee individuals rights against discrimination on the basis of race, sex, sexual orientation, religion, caste,

---

[5] These rights raise some questions about the nature and scope of punishment under care theory. For some discussions of care and punishment, see Noddings (2002: 265–82) and West (1997).

ethnicity, or national origin in matters directly affecting their ability to give or receive care. The logic for including this right among the list of caring rights is that discrimination can often threaten or impede individuals' abilities to care for themselves and others. When individuals cannot find remunerative work or housing because of their race or sex, their ability to care for themselves and their dependents will be seriously compromised. Where their sexual orientation or religion makes them public pariahs, their bodily health and integrity may be endangered. As such, antidiscrimination laws are a natural correlate of care theory. Care theory nonetheless does not necessarily support the extension of antidiscrimination rights to all areas of life or call for equal rights for all. If a private club wishes to exclude some group from membership and this club's decision has no impact on the group's ability to give and receive care, then care theory does not preclude discrimination in this case. The case against discrimination here would have to be made on the basis of equality, autonomy, utility, or some other value independent of care theory. Care theory supports antidiscrimination legislation only in matters that can be shown directly to impact individuals' abilities to care for themselves or others.

The first general task of a caring government may be summarized as providing individuals with public goods that they cannot easily obtain on their own and the basic rights necessary to ensure their security and ability to care for themselves and others. The second, and in many ways central, task of a caring government involves lending support to the inevitable dependencies of human life and the derivative dependencies that arise from caring for inevitably dependent individuals (Fineman 2004: 35–6). The inevitable dependencies of human life may be grouped into three broad categories: (a) infancy and childhood, (b) sickness and injury, and (c) frail old age and disability (Kittay 1999: 29). A caring government will ensure that inevitably dependent individuals are provided adequate care either by establishing programs to serve them directly or by offering subsidies and support to their primary caregivers.

In establishing caring programs, governments might justifiably use means testing to determine eligibility. We all have a moral obligation to help individuals in need, but not necessarily to help individuals who are capable of providing for themselves and their dependents by their own means. It is therefore morally legitimate within care theory to limit subsidies only to those individuals who cannot afford to care for themselves and their dependents. There are, however, some good moral and practical reasons for favoring universal, or at least nearly universal, programs over means-tested ones (Rothstein 1998: 144–70; Rothstein and Uslaner 2005). First, universal programs are easier and cheaper to administer and generally make caring services more accessible to all individuals since they do not require complicated eligibility requirements. Under universal programs, eligibility can be framed so simply (e.g. age) that it can be largely automated (Rothstein 1998: 160). Second, means-tested programs can be demeaning to people, especially when they are open only to the most desperately poor. These programs require individuals who may already feel ashamed of their lack of self-sufficiency to demonstrate their lack of self-sufficiency to government officials who may be suspicious of their claims. Some individuals who legitimately need care may therefore forego seeking it under means-tested programs. Third, means-tested programs may generate resentment among the rich and middle classes and make the poor feel that they stand apart from the rest of society, thus eroding a general sense of trust and solidarity among citizens that is important for maintaining social programs (Rothstein and Uslaner 2005). Finally, wealthy and middle class individuals may be less likely to show strong support for programs that offer them no benefits. Universal programs, by contrast, are more likely to enjoy strong support from all segments of society. Altogether, then, even though care theory recognizes the moral logic behind means testing, it generally favors universal programs whenever feasible. Means testing can have the unintended consequence of making social programs inaccessible and undermining broad and long-term support for caring policies. It might be possible, of course, to devise some sort of intermediate policy between fully universal programs and narrow means testing. Goods and services might be offered at graduated rates, for example, up to a fairly high income level. The challenge with these programs is to find an easy way to determine eligibility requirements without demeaning individuals who need care.

Returning now to care theory's substantive policy commitments, there are a number of steps a caring government might take to ensure the adequate care of infants and children. To begin with, all pregnant women should be guaranteed prenatal care and access to adequate nutrition. Basic prenatal care is important for identifying and addressing health problems that, if left untreated, may endanger the life or health of the pregnant woman and her fetus. Adequate nutrition is similarly important for pregnant women's health and fetal development. Iron, protein, and other sorts of deficiencies, for example, can result in stunted brain growth and permanent mental damage to the fetus (Administration for Children and Families 2001). Programs supporting accessible health care and nutrition for pregnant women thus represent the first plank of a caring program for children and their caregivers. *good leave*

Subsidized parental leaves represent a second important plank. All new parents should be guaranteed a certain amount of time off from work to care for their new infants and should be provided with a governmental subsidy during their leaves. The governmental subsidy is important so that all individuals have the opportunity actually to take advantage of these work leaves. Governments might alternatively require businesses to subsidize workers' leaves, but this would create a disincentive for businesses to hire workers likely to have children—especially young women. It would also unfairly burden particular businesses with the costs of supporting caregiving rather than evenly distributing these costs throughout society. There are thus some important advantages to subsidizing family leaves through public means.

The central justification for paid parental leaves derives from the importance of close personal care for infants during their first months of life. John Bowlby originally hypothesized an innate need among human infants for forming a secure attachment with one or more primary caregivers during the early months of their lives (Bowlby 1969, 1973, 1980). Infants specifically need to be able to rely upon one or more primary caregivers to meet their physical and emotional needs in sensitive and particular ways.[6] Bowlby argued that a secure attachment is essential for the normal physical, emotional, and mental development of children because it provides the basic framework through which children relate to others and the world around them for the rest of their lives. While certain aspects of Bowlby's hypothesis remain controversial, research has substantiated important parts of it (Fonagy 2001; Hrdy 1999; Siegel 1999: 67–120; Thompson 1998). Infants do seem to need, or at least greatly benefit from, the reliable presence of one or more primary caregivers during their early months. In *The Developing Mind*, Daniel Siegel writes that early secure attachment relationships 'are crucial in organizing not only ongoing experience, but the neuronal growth of the developing brain. In other words, these salient emotional relationships have a direct affect on the development of the domains of mental functioning that serve as our conceptual anchor points: memory, narrative, emotion, representations, and states of mind. In this way, attachment relationships may serve to create the central foundation from which the mind develops' (Siegel 1999:

[6] Bowlby originally suggested that infants particularly need the care of their mothers, but research has shown that infants can form secure attachments with a variety of different figures and may bond with more than one primary caregiver (Nussbaum 2001: 188).

83

68). Infants who form secure attachments with their primary caregivers tend to develop their emotional, cognitive, and social capabilities more quickly and fully than those who do not, while infants who do not form secure attachments tend to develop more slowly, have more difficulty regulating their emotions and behaviors, and are more prone to anxiety and aggression. Insecure attachments further create a significant risk of psychological and social dysfunction later in life (Siegel 1999: 68, 84). Research has also found a strong correlation between family leaves and substantial decreases in infant and early childhood mortality (Gornick and Meyers 2003: 242–3). The explanation for this finding is not entirely clear, but it may stem from the fact that new parents are more likely to provide more attentive, responsive, and respectful care to their new infants than others do. In general, then, a period of direct parental care seems a basic ingredient for ensuring adequate care for infants. While parental leaves surely cannot ensure that all infants will form a secure attachment with their primary caregivers, they do at least increase the likelihood that more infants will do so.

Just how much time off from work parents should be given and the amount of the subsidy are policy questions that must be decided by politicians, policymakers, and citizens. In European countries, where paid leaves are the norm, programs range from Switzerland's ten weeks of parental leave with wage replacement at a flat rate to Sweden's eighteen months of paid leave reimbursed at ninety percent of the leave-taker's pay (Gauthier 1996; Gornick and Meyers 2003: 112–46; Harrington 1999: 56; Cancian and Oliker 2000: 100–34). Since researchers have found that infants usually form attachments with their primary caregivers by about seven months, a seven-month leave would seem adequate (Siegel 1999: 68). Because parents will only take these leaves if they can afford to do so, the subsidy should further be set at a rate that makes parental leaves a real possibility for all new parents. The subsidy should also be made available to unemployed parents who may need support during the first months of their babies' lives so that they can care for their newborns without having to seek work or engage in job training.

Another important policy for supporting the adequate care of children involves providing income subsidies to families with children, especially poor families. Children of impoverished families are more likely to be undernourished, which can have long-term consequences for their cognitive development and health (Brown and Pollitt 1996; Rank 2004: 38–42). Childhood poverty further correlates with lower levels of physical and cognitive development, physical and mental health, school achievement, and adult employment (Rank 2004: 45; Streuning 2002: xvi). If we take seriously our obligation to help all individuals to develop their innate capabilities in adequate ways, we thus should recognize the duty to ensure that all families have the resources necessary to support adequate child development. These subsidies could be provided in easy and nonintrusive ways through government grants, tax rebates, and the like.

An objection may arise at this point (if not before) that parents should be responsible for providing for their own children. Other individuals should not be asked to subsidize the decisions of some individuals to have children; they should care for their own. The problem with this argument from the perspective of care theory is that it punishes children for their parents' choices. Children cannot be held responsible for the families that they are born into, and yet they depend upon their families to survive and develop. If their families cannot provide them with the care necessary to survive and develop in healthy and normal ways, then outside individuals are thus morally obligated to subsidize their care. Moreover, we all suffer at least indirectly when children receive inadequate care, since children who receive inadequate care are more likely to perform poorly in school, engage in crime and violence, abuse alcohol and drugs, have difficulty holding jobs and maintaining relationships, and suffer other difficulties (see below). Even if one may resent supporting other people's children (which a caring person will not do), one should be able to recognize the moral obligation and social importance of doing so.[7]

*TAKES A VILLAGE TO RAISE A CHILD?*

Public support for childcare represents another important element of a caring family policy. Because most people have to work outside the home to support themselves and their dependents, few parents are able to provide full-time personal care for their children. At the same time, few families can currently afford to purchase quality childcare in countries that do not publicly support it (Helburn and Bergmann 2002). As a result, many children in these countries receive poor quality childcare during their early years, which appears to have important long-term negative effects on their development and functioning. Children who receive inadequate childcare tend to develop more slowly and may suffer various emotional and health problems as they grow older (Blau 2001: 125–46; Helburn and Bergmann 2002: 55–85). Alternatively, children who are provided quality childcare and early education show long-term gains in academic achievement, emotional well-being, health, employment,

---

[7] Care theory does recognize a responsibility among individuals to try to have children only when they can care adequately for them. Any attempt to try to translate this personal responsibility into a law or policy, however, would almost surely have uncaring consequences.

and income, and are less likely to drop out of school, use drugs, engage in criminal activity, or remain unemployed for long periods (Campbell et al. 2002; Cubed 2002; Reynolds et al. 2001; Schweinhart 2004). In this respect, public childcare is not only a morally obligatory policy but also a cost-effective one. Quality childcare and early education programs for low-income children, in particular, have been estimated to save anywhere from $4 to $6 for every $1 spent by reducing special education, welfare, unemployment, and prison costs (Masse and Barnett 2002; Reynolds et al. 2001).[8] They further generate long-term higher tax revenues by increasing employment and productivity. Taking into account both the reductions in public expenditures and increased revenues from taxes, one recent study *conservatively* estimates that investments in quality childcare programs generate an overall return to society of $17 for each $1 invested (Schweinhart 2004).[9]

There are a variety of possibilities for publicly supporting quality childcare (Albelda 2004; Bergmann 2004; Gornick and Meyers 2003: 185–235; Koren 2004). The French government provides free high quality nursery schools/childcare centers for all children from ages 3 to 5 (Folbre 2001: 132–4). Eva Kittay proposes a direct public subsidy for parents that they could use to support themselves while caring for their children or to purchase quality childcare (1999: 143).[10] Various plans also exist for subsidizing quality childcare through private providers (Blau 2001: 208–32; Helburn and Bergmann 2002). Suzanne Helburn and Barbara Bergmann have outlined one plan that requires parents to pay no more than twenty percent of their above poverty-level income for quality childcare and early education services, with the government subsidizing the remaining costs and enforcing quality-control measures (Helburn and Bergmann 2002: 15–32). Under this plan, the poorest families would pay nothing for quality childcare and partial subsidies would be extended at graduated levels to families well above the median income level—up to $76,845 in current US dollars (29). Whether a society prefers a system of publicly funded childcare and early education centers, direct subsidies to parents, subsidies for childcare and early education centers, or some other arrangement is once again a policy decision depending in part upon people's priorities. Because women are most likely to use long-term direct

---

[8] See also the Carolina Abecedarian Project (www.fpg.unc.edu/~abc/).

[9] See also L. J. Schweinhart et al. (2005) and Kirp (2004).

[10] Alstott outlines a similar proposal, but in her plan parents could also use the subsidy to pay for their own education or place it in a retirement account. Her policy proposal is guided primarily by the aim of providing parents with more autonomy and choice rather than guaranteeing children adequate care (2004: 110–11).

parenting subsidies, these subsidies tend to strengthen traditional family arrangements but reduce gender equality. Public childcare arrangements, by contrast, tend to promote greater gender equality, but offer parents less flexibility in determining how to care for their children. While care theory generally remains open toward different childcare policies, it does nevertheless offer two guidelines in deciding between different programs. First, a good case can be made for encouraging parents to enroll their children in childcare and early education centers at least at age three or four in order to foster their early development and ensure quality care (Helburn and Bergmann 2002: 49–52).[11] Second, programs should be designed in a manner that allows childcare centers some flexibility in responding to their clients' needs and provides parents some flexibility over their childcare arrangements.

A caring government should finally guarantee all children an education sufficient to develop their basic capabilities for emotion, language, imagination, reason, affiliation, reading, writing, and math. All children need education in order to develop their basic capabilities, but few parents have the time and ability on their own to prepare their children adequately for successful social functioning in a complex industrial society. Education is also a public good that benefits many individuals regardless of their contribution to it. Thus, a caring government will make some sort of public provision to ensure that all children have access to adequate education. Governments might adopt a variety of different plans for publicly supporting education, including directly establishing and maintaining a public education system or providing parents with education vouchers to pay for their children's education. Any of a number of plans might be consistent with the aims of care theory. It is important, however, to be clear about these aims. Care theory supports a broad fundamentals education that aims to help children to develop not only their intellectual capabilities but also their emotional, imaginative, and social potentialities. A focus on reading, math, and other cognitive skills is important, but should not be allowed to push out programs in the arts and other subjects essential for developing the full range of children's innate capabilities.[12] Since the development of children's innate capabilities generally entails a great deal of personal attention, care theory further supports small class sizes and low teacher–student ratios. From a caring perspective, the

[11] This point will be further discussed in Chapter 5.
[12] In Chapter 5, I discuss a caring education program in more detail.

adequacy of different education plans can ultimately be measured by their success in meeting these goals.

The second inevitable dependency covered by a caring government is sickness and injury. We all suffer illnesses or injuries at some time in our lives that require medical and personal care to restore our health or ease our pain. Governments can help us to cope with these periods of inevitable need by guaranteeing long-term subsidized sick leaves from work for individuals with serious illnesses or injuries, and subsidized caretaker leaves for individuals to care for sick or injured dependents. Governments can also mandate a number of sick days from work each year for workers so that they can care for themselves and their dependents as necessary. Beyond these policies, governments should further guarantee all individuals access to adequate medical care. With regard to medical care, a difficult question arises about what exactly should count as adequate. Given our duty to care for individuals in need, we should do all that we can to improve the health and prolong the lives of all individuals who wish to continue living. Yet the development of ever new and more expensive medical technologies means the pursuit of this goal could lead to excessive health care costs. Much of a society's resources could be eaten up in attempting to provide every individual with every new treatment or technology. Care theory avoids this untenable outcome by situating our need for health care in the context of an overall care framework. While health care is an extremely important good, it should not be allowed to overshadow people's need for various other forms of care or the other goods that they might wish to pursue. In this regard, adequate medical care might be defined as access to all the medical goods, services, and technologies necessary for survival, health, and functioning *given available social resources.*

In the United States, most individuals currently purchase health care insurance privately or acquire it through their place of employment. This method of distributing health care services is clearly inadequate. Despite spending more than twice as much per capita on health care than any other country, the United States has shorter life spans, lower patient satisfaction, and more intrusion into clinical decisions than nearly every country with a universal health care system (Kuttner 1997: 155; Rank 2004: 211). Moreover, more than forty million Americans have no health insurance and many more are underinsured.

The Physicians' Working Group for Single-Payer National Health Insurance has outlined one plan for addressing these problems (2003). Their national health insurance plan would cover every American for all medically necessary services, including doctor's visits, necessary operations, prenatal care, long-term care, mental health and dental services, and prescription drugs and supplies. By eliminating the high administrative costs, profits, and advertising expenses of private insurance companies, this plan would save at least $200 billion annually, which is more than enough to offset the expenses of universal coverage. Additional savings would likely come from the better health of all citizens, and decreased reliance among the uninsured upon catastrophic and emergency room care. The plan would therefore require no additional expenses beyond what individuals and companies currently pay for health insurance— that is, existing levels of socially available resources. Individuals and businesses would simply pay the government instead of private insurers for their health insurance coverage.[13] Since overall expenditures would remain at current levels, this plan would avoid many of the problems associated with other universal health care systems, (e.g. the Canadian system) whose flaws stem mainly from inadequate funding rather than the single-payer format. Individuals would also still be free under this plan—or actually freer than many Americans currently are under their HMO plans—to seek care from any licensed care professional.

The Physicians' Working Group Plan represents only one cost-efficient way to ensure adequate health care for all individuals; other plans might also be acceptable. In the United States, for example, the government could vastly expand the Medicaid program to cover all unemployed individuals while requiring all businesses to provide insurance coverage to their employees, or offer subsidies to low-income individuals so that they could purchase their health care from private providers. There are, however, some drawbacks to these proposals: they are unlikely to contain medical costs as effectively as a national system or to provide as high a level of health care to all individuals, and once again they unfairly burden businesses with the costs of paying for their employees' care. Care theory nonetheless remains flexible and pragmatic on health care policy just as it does on other policy matters. What matters is that all individuals have access to adequate medical care.

The third category of inevitable dependencies is frail old age and disability. There are many elderly and disabled individuals who have no acute medical problems but whose quality of life is dependent upon the

---

[13] How exactly taxes would be leveled for this program—on individuals, businesses, etc.—is once again a policy question. The point I am making here is simply that the program would not cost any more than the government, businesses, and individuals in the United States currently spend on health care.

long-term care of others. With periodic home visits from care workers and other social-support services (housekeeping, transportation), many of these individuals can maintain independent living arrangements and for the most part care for themselves (Clement 1996: 98). A caring government would provide or subsidize these sorts of care services as well as more institutionalized forms of care such as nursing homes for individuals who prefer or require them. It would further provide income support and social services to parents whose children require permanent intensive personal care due to a disability, as well as to other individuals who are responsible for the long-term intensive care of an elderly or disabled person.[14]

Public subsidies should also be provided for the basic needs of the frail elderly, disabled, and other individuals who cannot work or otherwise provide for themselves. In the United States, old age and disability subsidies are currently provided through the social security system. While predictions of social security's demise appear to be premature, some reforms may be necessary to sustain this system, and care theory offers some guidance in this regard (Baker and Weisbrot 2001; Gordon 2003). At present, social security is framed primarily as a sort of public pension program that returns to individuals some portion of the income they contribute into it over the course of their lives. From the perspective of care theory, it seems reasonable to reframe the philosophy and objectives of this program. In the first place, social security might be reformulated as a social subsidy program that offers all elderly, disabled, and other individuals in need an adequate basic income. Individuals who earned high incomes throughout their lives would receive the same basic subsidy under this plan as individuals who earned lower incomes. Meanwhile, incentives in the form of tax breaks for retirement accounts and other measures might be offered to encourage individuals to save additional money for their retirement. The age at which elderly individuals might begin receiving social security benefits might also be raised slightly (with special exceptions for those who need support at younger ages). The goal of an old-age subsidy program under care theory should be to provide for the frail elderly who can no longer support themselves rather than to subsidize the early retirement of still capable elderly persons. Finally, the social security tax might also be raised on high income earners. At present in the United States, the social security tax is capped at $94,400. The cap seems arbitrary and unjust given that high-income earners are generally

---

[14] Anne Alstott outlines a plan for helping parents of ill or disabled children (2004: 117–37). Her program might be extended to other individuals who take on the intensive and long-term care of elderly individuals and others.

more capable than others of contributing to the care of frail elderly and disabled individuals.

It might be questioned here why children should not be primarily responsible for the care of their frail elderly parents rather than shifting the burden to society as a whole. A moment's reflection should suffice for an answer. In modern industrialized societies, many children no longer live in close proximity to their parents, enjoy close relations with them, or have the time or energy to care for them personally without some sort of assistance. Most elderly individuals, in turn, prefer governmental support over reliance upon their children or other family members, in part because they do not wish to be a burden to them (Goodin 1988: 350–1). As with the care of children, then, if we wish to guarantee all frail elderly individuals adequate care (as we should), there are good reasons for providing public services and support to them.

Besides providing support for the inevitable dependencies of human life, a caring government will also provide residual support to capable individuals who cannot care adequately for themselves and their dependents despite making reasonable efforts to do so. Even in a safe and prosperous social environment, some capable individuals may not be able to satisfy their basic needs at minimally adequate levels, perhaps because of a shortage of decent paying jobs or affordable housing. Some individuals may also require temporary assistance due to unemployment or some other hardship. A caring government will step in to help these individuals with income supplements or other forms of support (e.g. housing vouchers) so that they can meet their basic needs and maintain at least a basic level of well-being. As argued in Chapter 1, individuals do have a responsibility under care theory to provide as much as possible for themselves and their dependents. As such, residual support for individuals might be made contingent upon their working, actively seeking work, taking part in a job training program, attending college, or caring for others. In any case, a caring government will provide residual support for individuals who cannot reasonably support themselves in the form of public subsidies, tax credits, unemployment insurance, or vouchers for basic goods. These and other programs related to the economy and employment will be further discussed in Chapter 3.

Care theory finally requires that governments remain attentive, responsive, and respectful toward the people within their jurisdictions. Attentiveness, responsiveness, and respect are no less important in caring at the institutional level than they are in caring at the personal level. Unless government officials are aware of what people need, monitor the effectiveness of caring programs, and involve people in the implementation and design of these programs, they are unlikely to care effectively for them. Joan Tronto has argued in this regard that care theory is most compatible with liberal democratic institutions. By her account, liberal democratic institutions constitute a part of care because they promote listening and responding and allow citizens to express and discuss their needs (Tronto 1993: 157–80). While there is some plausibility to Tronto's position, the link between care theory and liberal democracy is looser than she suggests. On the one hand, liberal democratic institutions are not sufficient to ensure attentiveness, responsiveness, and respect. Liberal democratic governments generally attend and respond to majority demands and interest group pressures, but are not always sensitive to the basic needs of all citizens, especially the poor and disenfranchised. On the other hand, liberal democratic institutions are also not necessary for governmental attentiveness, responsiveness, and respect. It is at least possible to imagine a nonliberal, nondemocratic form of government (e.g. a 'parliament of scholars' or publicly oriented merit-based bureaucracy) that would be highly attentive, responsive, and respectful to people and their needs (Bell 2000: 279–336). In some cases, governments might actually be more attentive and responsive to the needs of all individuals if they were somewhat insulated from the pressures of democratic and interest group politics.

One argument apparently supporting Tronto's position is Amatya Sen's claim that no substantial famine has ever occurred in any country with a democratic form of government (Sen 1999: 160–88). Sen's argument has sometimes been taken to mean that liberal democracies are practically more attentive and responsive to people's needs than other forms of government. As Sen himself notes, however, while liberal democracies are better than most other forms of government in avoiding large-scale crises, they are not necessarily better at guaranteeing the everyday needs of people or eliminating problems such as malnutrition (Sen 1999: 154, 160–61). Other governmental arrangements may actually be better at satisfying the basic biological and developmental needs of people than liberal democracies are.

None of this should be taken to mean that care theory is opposed to liberal democratic institutions. Liberal democracies do appear on average to be less likely to harm people and more likely to attend and respond to majority interests than most other forms of government. Moreover, some measure of freedom of speech and the press is important for providing people with an opportunity to express their needs and preferences to government officials. In this regard, care theory might be said to show a slight on average preference for liberal democratic institutions. But care theory cannot be said definitively to endorse or require this form of government. Rather, the criterion for judging the legitimacy of any form of government from the perspective of care theory is whether it is attentive and responsive to people's needs and effective at helping them to meet them. In different countries or cultures, different sorts of governmental arrangements might be best suited for meeting this goal. In the final analysis, the general form of government (democracy, theocracy, or aristocracy) is less important for care theory than the mode of the government's administration. In order to remain attentive, responsive, and respectful toward people, governments need to engage people at local levels in the implementation and design of policies (principle 4 above), shift the delivery of care as much as possible to local levels (principle 5), and reach out to ensure that support services are known and accessible to all people (principle 6). While care theory does not require democracy at the macrolevel, it does require flexible and decentralized social programs and some measure of democracy at local levels.

## 2.4. Just Another Welfare State?

The principles, institutions, and policies of a caring government resemble in many ways those of traditional liberal welfare states. Yet to conflate care theory with welfare liberalism is to miss much that is new and innovative about care theory. Liberal welfare states emerged in a piecemeal fashion during the nineteenth and twentieth centuries largely in response to the social crises and movements of the time. In the process, welfare policies were grafted onto a classical liberal framework that is not especially well suited for supporting them (Goodin 1988). Donald Moon writes, for example, that the liberal principle of individual autonomy 'poses a serious dilemma for a polity that aspires to be a welfare state. For if people hold the norm that they should be independent (in the sense of self-supporting), then how can the state provide them with the means of subsistence without violating their self-respect?' (Moon 1988: 35). Other theorists have similarly noted that the classical liberal ideals of individual freedom and autonomy tend to stigmatize dependency and welfare (Fraser and Gordon 2002; Young 2002). While there are some sound liberal justifications for traditional welfare policies, the liberal ideology offers

93

equally sound justifications for opposing these policies.[15] As a result, the liberal welfare state has always been riddled with ambiguities and tensions that have contributed in part to the sometimes inconsistent, begrudging, and haphazard implementation of social programs.

Care theory offers a more cogent framework for supporting caring welfare policies. Starting out from the premise of human dependency, care theory suggests that government should help individuals to meet their biological and developmental needs in all those areas of life and circumstances where they cannot reasonably meet their needs on their own. It thus provides more cogent support for many welfare—and especially caring—policies than liberalism can supply.

The aims of a caring government are also notably different from the aims of most liberal welfare states. Liberal welfare states have traditionally aimed to buffer individuals against market uncertainties and failures by providing unemployment insurance, disability pensions, and other safety net measures. They have tended to regard caring practices, however, as primarily a private responsibility outside the public sphere.[16] A caring government, by contrast, makes support and accommodation of caring activities its central focus. It organizes programs to support caregivers and ensure that all individuals receive the care they need during periods of inevitable dependency and dire need. In doing so, it recasts the central purpose behind most state assistance programs. Many liberal welfare programs provide support for individuals only after they have lost their jobs, suffered an injury, or become incapable of working. Care theory supports these traditional sorts of welfare programs, but more generally supports proactive policies that are likely to reduce the need for traditional forms of welfare. As noted above, for example, quality childcare and early education programs lead to higher academic achievement, lower drop-out rates, increased earning power, reduced levels of criminal activity, less dependence on welfare, and reduced risks of poverty (Campbell et al. 2002; Cubed 2002; Reynolds et al. 2001; Schweinhart 2004). By investing in these sorts of programs, a caring government minimizes the long-term need for unemployment insurance, income subsidies, and other traditional liberal welfare programs—as well as more police, judges, and

---

[15] Stephen Holmes (1988) argues against libertarian writers that the liberal tradition contains principles of social responsibility and wealth distribution. While his point is well taken, the principles of social responsibility in liberalism at least stand in tension with the tradition's clear commitment to individual liberty and property rights.

[16] Since World War II, many European states have introduced programs to support personal caring, but the theory and justification for these new-style welfare states remains underdeveloped. Care theory provides such a theory and justification.

prisons. It gives more emphasis to enabling and preventative policies so that traditional welfare policies will become less necessary. Jean Gardiner has suggested in this regard that a caring government is better understood as a developmental state than a welfare state (Gardiner 1997). It takes an active role in helping people to develop and sustain (as much as they are able) their innate capabilities and social functioning rather than focusing primarily—as, for example, Rawls's liberal welfare theory does—on redistributing income and alleviating poverty.

A caring government finally departs from the theory and practice of traditional welfare states in its greater attention to the manner of providing goods and services to individuals. Most welfare states and welfare state theories are concerned primarily with the distribution of goods, but show little concern for how these goods are provided. Some of the worst missteps of traditional welfare states have stemmed from this myopia. Programs have been designed and implemented without careful attention to the people they are supposed to serve. Predictably enough, many of these programs have failed to achieve their goals and some have even exacerbated social problems (White 2000). Care theory emphasizes the importance of providing goods and services in a caring manner. This means involving potential care recipients in the design and implementation of programs whenever possible, and supporting family and personal caring in a flexible and decentralized manner. By practicing these policies, a caring government further avoids one of the most long-standing and decisive criticisms of welfare programs: that they weaken civil society and breed apathy among people. A caring government supports some of the central institutions of civil society, including families, childcare centers, schools, and community groups, and further facilitates civic engagement by involving people in local program design and implementation.

## 2.5. Care Theory and Multiculturalism

In recent years, political theorists have become much more sensitive to issues of multicultural justice. Since most societies are populated by people holding diverse cultural, religious, and moral values, most theorists have come to recognize the need to consider these different values in outlining their theories of justice (Benhabib 2002; Fraser and Honneth 2003; Kymlicka 1995; Parekh 2000; Rawls 1996; Taylor 1994; Valadez 2001; Young 1990). Care theory intersects with questions of multicultural justice in important and intimate ways. Many (but certainly not all)

clashes over multiculturalism involve questions about caring for children, the sick, and others. Any complete account of a caring theory of justice thus must confront questions of multicultural justice. Somewhat surprisingly, though, care theorists have generally had very little to say about this important issue.

On the most general level, care theory can be said to endorse tolerance toward many personal multicultural practices and traditions. A caring government will not require all groups and individuals to care for dependents in exactly the same way but allows for a fair amount of diversity in meeting needs and fostering capabilities. Since caring is usually provided most effectively in close personal relations, a caring government will generally not intrude upon personal caring relations or local care arrangements but permit individuals a good deal of leeway in caring for their loved ones. A government that too closely monitors personal care or attempts to dictate too precise standards for caring relations is likely to undermine rather than encourage good care. Even personal caring practices that are suboptimal should generally be tolerated, since the disruption caused by government intervention into family and personal relationships can often make matters worse (Alstott 2004: 42–3). The only constraint a caring government will place upon caregivers is that they must meet the biological and developmental needs of their dependents at least at adequate threshold levels. As long as caregivers meet this requirement, a caring government will generally leave them alone to care as they see fit.

This last stipulation, however, is where conflicts are likely to arise. If a government is to ensure the adequate care of all individuals, it must define some minimal standards of adequate care. Yet different cultural and religious groups may have very different ideas about what constitutes minimally adequate parental, medical, or other forms of care. Different societies, for example, define child abuse and neglect quite differently (Korbin 1977, 1979, 1981, 1982). Western people often look upon initiation rites in other cultures such as female genital operations and ritual scarification as abusive, while non-Western people frequently view Western parenting practice as neglectful. The cultural anthropologist Jill Korbin writes:

Non-western peoples often conclude that the anthropologists, missionaries, and other Europeans with whom they come into contact at best do not know how to rear children and, at worst, simply do not love their offspring. Practices such as isolating children in rooms of their own at night, making infants wait a given number of hours to be fed, or allowing small children to 'cry themselves out' would be at odds with the child-rearing philosophies of many cultures. (Korbin 1982: 259)

How, then, should child abuse and neglect be defined? In a similar vein, while some standards can be specified for adequate medical care based upon Western medical practices, not everyone regards Western medical technology as an appropriate standard for adequate health care. Christian Scientists, for example, view disease as an illusion created by God and best treated through faith healing. In their view, seeking medical help under-mines the effectiveness of faith healing (Renteln 2004: 65). Should, then, Christian Scientists be allowed to reject medical care for their children on the grounds that they consider faith healing to represent the best form of care? Different groups may also have different ideas about the value and purpose of education. In the United States, for example, the Amish have won the right to withdraw their children from public education at age 14 in order to teach them the skills of farming and domestic labor and preserve their traditional religious lifestyle. Does this constitute a minimally adequate education?

In addressing these questions, it first needs to be considered whether caring practices can be separated out from their cultural expression or whether caring is so saturated with cultural meaning that it offers no independent standpoint from which to assess cultural practices. As noted in Chapter 1, if we define caring in terms of the particular practices of different groups, then caring would not seem to be able to provide any sort of cross-cultural standard. Different groups care for the young, sick, elderly, disabled, and needy in very different ways (Collins 2000; Hays 1996; Korbin, 1981; Kurtz 1992; Liederman, Tulkin, and Rosenfeld 1977; Renteln 2004). If, however, caring is defined more generally as everything we do directly to help individuals to meet their basic biological and devel-opmental needs, then it has a more universal application. All cultures and groups necessarily engage in practices of caring that help individuals to meet their basic biological and developmental needs. Any culture or group that did not engage in such practices would not exist for very long. A generic structural definition of caring can therefore be separated out from its cultural manifestations. Those practices within a people's culture that aim directly to meet the basic biological or developmental needs of individuals may be defined as caring, and those practices that have other aims pertain to other aspects of their culture.

Care theory privileges the generic structural aims of caring practices over cultural and religious customs and beliefs that may influence their particular expression. It does so on the grounds that all cultures and religions depend upon generic caring practices to ensure the survival, development, and functioning of their members. If no one cared for others in the generic sense of helping them to meet their biological and developmental needs, there would be no individuals or societies and hence no cultures or religions. Cultural or religious practices that impede or contravene the generic aims of caring are therefore contradictory. While they rely upon generic caring practices for their existence, they ignore or subvert the aims of these practices for other goals. Even if these cultures or religions may be able to perpetuate themselves while denying adequate care to some individuals, they necessarily involve the individuals who support them in a performative contradiction. Since individuals generally desire survival and functioning, appeal to others for the care necessary to achieve these aims, and thus commit themselves to the general moral principle that capable individuals should care for individuals in need, they cannot support cultures or religions that impede the care of others without contradicting their own implicit moral beliefs—that is, the belief that capable individuals should care for others in need and help them achieve social functioning.

The morality of different cultural and religious practices can therefore be judged by considering whether they effectively satisfy—or at least do not impede the satisfaction of—individuals' needs for nutritious food, sanitary water, protective shelter, education, and the like. Practices that effectively support adequate care for all individuals are moral, practices that impede adequate care are immoral, and practices that neither support nor impede adequate care are indifferent. Practices that a group may call caring but nonetheless fail to meet the basic biological and developmental needs of individuals are not less contradictory just because a group dubs them as caring, but rather doubly flawed. They not only fail to satisfy the generic aims of caring but in most cases fail even to meet the group's own self-ascribed goals for them. A group whose eating habits fail to nourish the young, for example, does not satisfy even its own goal of adequately feeding these individuals, and a group whose healing practices fail to cure illnesses and alleviate pain does not satisfy the purpose for which healing practices usually exist. The generic aims of caring thus provide a pragmatic standard by which the morality of different customs and practices can be measured. The morality of different 'caring' customs and practices can be determined by 'cashing them out' to see if they actually meet the generic aims of caring (James 1991).

Care theory privileges not only the generic features of caring over cultural values, but also the care of individuals over group values and goals. We all claim care from others as individuals, and in fact it is our very dependency *as individuals* that draws us together into groups. As such, we all have an obligation to care for other individuals in need over and above group values or goals, or at least to ensure that group values or goals guarantee adequate care to all individuals. It is hypocritical and contradictory from the perspective of care theory for individuals to place group or cultural values above the basic care of individuals when our own claims for care are necessarily individual in nature. While individuals certainly could not survive without the group, we are born into the group as individually embodied beings and it is as individually embodied beings that we claim and receive care. It is therefore to individuals that we owe care. The group exists in care theory to support individuals and not the other way around. Care theory's notion of interdependency can be contrasted in this regard with the idea of collectivism: interdependency recognizes the dependency of individuals upon one another for care, and supports a theory of community and politics resting upon caring relationships. Collectivism, by contrast, subordinates individuals to an already existent and usually abstract ideal of community.

The moral priority that care theory gives to individuals should not be taken to mean that individuals would be wrong in their own lives to place group values over their own care. Competent and capable adults always retain the right to waive off offers of caring in order to pursue other values or goals. They do not, however, possess the right to deny others care, and even in their own cases, they should at least have access to the goods and services necessary to care adequately for themselves if they should choose to do so. Any group that denies some individuals even the opportunity to give or receive adequate care holds some highly questionable, and ultimately immoral, values.

Care theory's general approach to culture, religion, and group values can be exemplified by outlining its approach to the oppression of women. Many societies limit women's access to social opportunities, resources, and other goods on the grounds that they are in some way inferior to men or need special protections, or in order to ensure their continued commitment to performing the care work of society. If women were to be offered more opportunities to work outside the home, more choice over their marriage partners, and more opportunity to care for themselves, then (the thinking goes) they would be less likely to devote themselves as diligently to the care of their children, husbands, and sick and elderly relations, and the overall quality of caring throughout society would suffer.

Care theory challenges these arrangements by cashing out their effects on women's survival, development, and basic social functioning. As argued in Chapter 1, we all have a moral duty to ensure to the best of our abilities that all individuals have the opportunity to give and receive decent care. Yet, when women are deprived of resources, opportunities, and other social goods, their ability to care for themselves and others is in most cases greatly compromised. At the very least, they are made more vulnerable to domestic violence and abuse because of their extreme dependency upon their husbands, fathers, and other men for the resources necessary to care for themselves and their children, parents, siblings, and other dependents (Okin 1989a). If their husbands or fathers should die or cast them out of their homes, they are further unlikely to be able to support themselves and their dependents. Where women lack access to social opportunities and resources, their lives are also likely to be devalued, as attested by Amartya Sen's index of the millions of missing women (Sen 1999: 104–7). Because girls are viewed as a burden on their families in countries where they enjoy few social opportunities, they tend to receive fewer resources and less attention, and hence die in far greater numbers. Given these considerations, oppressive social practices toward women may be said to be generally uncaring (even when ostensibly justified by caring goals) on the grounds that they sacrifice the care of some individuals for the care of others. Based upon the moral framework developed in Chapter 1, no one should be forced to sacrifice self-care for the care of others or have their right to adequate care ignored. It nonetheless should be noted that adequate care for women can be secured in many cultures under conditions of less than full social and political equality. Care theory favors the lifting of oppressive practices only so far as they are necessary to ensure adequate care for all individuals, but does not necessarily favor full social or political equality for all. Full social and political equality is a liberal value that can supplement care theory but does not find support within it.

Most cultures and religions do, of course, contain general dictates in support of caring values and practices. All of the world's major religions, for example, have core teachings about the duty to care for others in need (Lauren 1998: 15–19). Most major moral systems likewise emphasize our moral duties to help the sick, injured, young, disabled, and otherwise needy. In most cases, then, deep conflicts between the principles of care theory and comprehensive religious and moral doctrines can be averted.

Individuals or groups who support uncaring practices can usually be shown to be out of step not only with the moral principle of caring but also with some of the core doctrines of their own religious or moral system. Even in cultures that do not support women's equality, for example, many oppressive practices can be challenged on the grounds that they impede women's survival and functioning and fail to show them the basic compassion and care that their own religious, cultural, or moral beliefs call for.

Most individuals or groups who support apparently uncaring practices can therefore be engaged under care theory in a process of cross-cultural dialogue. Individuals who favor practices that apparently deprive some people of access to their basic needs can be asked to explain why they support these practices. In some cases, they may explain that the apparently uncaring practices are not actually uncaring when considered in their societal or cultural context—perhaps because they are balanced out by other forms of social support. In other cases, individuals may be challenged to rethink their cultural beliefs or practices because of their effects on individual caring. Care theory favors this sort of cross-cultural dialogue because hasty judgments about another group's practices fail to show the individuals within these groups the attentiveness, responsiveness, and respect that is central to caring. Moreover, hasty judgments may overlook the ways in which the bundles of goods and services provided to individuals in a given group may compensate for particular goods and services that are not offered to all individuals (Sen 1984: 513–4).

Care theory's approach to multiculturalism overlaps in this regard with the views of advocates of deliberative democracy who have argued that free and open debate represents the only fair way to reach some sort of resolution on questions of multicultural justice (Benhabib 2002; Parekh 2000; Valadez 2001). Bhikhu Parekh summarizes his approach to cross-cultural dialogue in the following way:

Rather than use the operative public values as a crude and non-negotiable standard for evaluating minority practices, society should engage in a dialogue with the minority. Since it disapproves of the minority practice, it needs to give reasons, and that involves showing why it holds these values and how the minority practice offends against them. For its part the minority needs to show why it follows the practice and offer a defence of it. (2000: 270)

Care theory endorses this model of cross-cultural dialogue, but with the further stipulation that discussions about the morality of different practices should revolve around the substantive issue of caring. Because all individuals depend upon the care of others for their survival and functioning, and most religious, moral, and cultural systems recognize the value of caring for others as a fundamental good, most individuals should be willing to accept adequate care as a common standard for assessing the morality of different cultural practices. If we can all agree (as we should be able to do given our common dependency) that it is morally good whenever possible to help individuals to meet their needs for food, water, shelter, education, medical care, and the like, then we can all be said to share some common goals for discussing a minimal basic morality. We can therefore justifiably ask one another to demonstrate empirically how a given practice serves to meet the basic needs of individuals. Reasonable individuals should be able to recognize the moral failings of any practices that prevent any individuals from adequately satisfying their vital biological and developmental needs. As a practical matter, of course, some individuals may not be willing to admit the shortcomings of their practices or beliefs. But care theory at least provides some grounds for assessing different practices that can be shown on rational grounds to be moral, and that most people should be willing to acknowledge as important human and social values.

Governments are ultimately responsible for defining and enforcing standards of minimally adequate care within their jurisdictions. It is not that government officials hold any sort of monopoly on the proper definition of caring; on the contrary, definitions of adequate care are always open to contestation and revision. Citizens, public officials, human rights advocates, foreign governments, and other individuals and groups may always challenge a government's definition of adequate care. However, if governments are going to fulfill their role in facilitating and enforcing adequate care within their jurisdictions, they must stipulate some standards of adequate care. In defining these standards, governments should consider the requirements of human survival, development, and basic functioning in their societies. As long as individuals and groups meet these goals, they should be left alone—and provided with the various forms of public support discussed above—to feed, clothe, shelter, and otherwise care for their children and other dependents as they think best. If individuals or groups fail to meet these goals, they should be engaged in the sort of cross-cultural dialogue about caring discussed above, and if necessary, forced to provide adequate care to all individuals.

Ayelet Shachar criticizes this approach to multicultural justice on the grounds that cultural groups may still be subjected to the arbitrary standards and decisions of government officials. 'We must be concerned with how "minimal standards" will be defined. We must also ask who will define them, and how' (2001: 111). In the past, for example, government officials in the United States have removed Native American children from their natural parents even though the officials had 'no basis for intelligently evaluating the cultural and social premises underlying Indian home life and child rearing' (111). While Shachar raises an important concern, the problem in this case seems to have stemmed from an overly narrow definition of adequate child rearing and a failure of cross-cultural dialogue. As long as parents are meeting their children's basic needs and helping them to achieve basic functioning, governments should not forcefully intrude into their lives. Where parents or other caregivers appear to be providing inadequate care, they should be engaged in cross-cultural dialogue about the nature and goals of their caring. If children are being neglected or harmed, then there would seem to be good grounds for removing them from their homes. The underlying approach here is pragmatic and consequentialist. Governments should assess the adequacy of caring practices not by judging their form but rather by evaluating their actual or probable results on the health, safety, and development of children and other dependents.

Having laid out a general framework for care theory and multiculturalism, we may now return to address the specific questions of multicultural justice raised at the beginning of this section. Regarding the abuse and neglect of children, care theory draws the line at any practice that threatens children's survival or health, damages their long-term physical and emotional development, or causes them unnecessary suffering or pain. Given these criteria, severe beatings are always wrong—even when justified on cultural grounds—because they can pose grave dangers to children's survival and health, may damage their development, and expose them to unnecessary pain and suffering. Intrusive initiation rites such as female genital cutting are unacceptable for similar reasons. These operations represent violations of girls' bodily integrity, impede their sensory development, and often result in threats to their survival and health (Williams 2000: 264).[17] The morality of other practices such as ritual scarring or tattooing are more open to debate and depend in large part upon the social context in which they occur. Since these practices generally do not represent serious threats to the survival or health of children or significantly impede the development of their basic

---

[17] Strategies for dealing with female circumcision and other apparently uncaring practices in other countries will be further discussed in Chapter 4.

103

capabilities, they cannot be ruled out on these grounds. The pain caused by these procedures can further be justified as warranted in societies where ritual markings help a person to secure a place in society and facilitate social functioning. For individuals who live outside of cultures that practice ritual scarring or tattooing, however, these practices may be said to cause unwarranted pain and may impede their ability to function in society. Thus Western governments would be justified in outlawing ritual scarring and tattooing of children within their jurisdictions but might nonetheless recognize the legitimacy of these practices in foreign cultures where they are the norm.[18] The morality of a number of other practices such as spanking, male circumcision, and ear and body piercing of children are further open to debate. Different people might reasonably disagree about whether the pain caused by these practices is acceptable. Where care theory clearly draws the line is at any practice that threatens the survival, development, health, or functioning of a child. Since Western childrearing practices such as placing infants in a separate room to sleep or feeding them at regular times generally do not appear to affect the survival, development, or health of children, these practices are acceptable—despite the horror they provoke in many non-Western mothers and regardless of whether they are optimal.

Care theory adopts a similarly pragmatic and consequentialist approach toward assessing the morality of different medical and healing practices. While different cultures may embrace a diversity of healing practices, they all ultimately share the same basic goal of promoting the good health of individuals and alleviating their pain and suffering. Any medical practices that are reasonably successful in achieving these goals are acceptable by the standards of care theory. As long, then, as Christian Scientist parents are able to maintain the health and functioning of their children through faith healing, the government would be unjustified in interfering in the care of their children. The government should further look seriously into the claim made by Christian Scientists that their faith-based methods of health care are every bit as effective as medical care. If this claim proves to be true, then government interference would likewise be unjustified. But if the Christian Scientists' claims cannot be persuasively demonstrated and modern medical technology can be shown to be more effective in treating various illnesses, then the government should intervene to provide the children of Christian Scientist parents with access to modern medical

---

[18] Renteln notes that the practice of scarification appears to be dying out except in remote areas, making its defensibility even in these areas increasing suspect (Renteln 2004: 51).

technology. Just as a person on a beach would be morally obligated to save a drowning child whose parents adopted some unorthodox and apparently ineffective method for saving him or her, a caring government is morally responsible for assuming direct care for the medical treatment of children whose parents' methods do not appear to be working.

Since the failure of caring in this case is limited only to medical issues, there is no need for the government to remove these children entirely from their parents. Instead, it might require only that Christian Scientist parents report to a social worker when their child is seriously ill and allow the social worker to take the child to a doctor if necessary.[19] The government might also mandate periodic health screenings of Christian Scientist (and, in fact, all) children to test for diabetes and other treatable illnesses. These policies obviously conflict with core beliefs of Christian Scientist parents and even their sense of what it means to provide good care to their children. The obligation to care for others, however, commits us to do what we can to care for children and other dependent individuals in light of demonstrably effective methods of caring. Just because a group claims that some practice is caring does not necessarily make it so.

An important distinction should nonetheless be drawn here between the care of adults and children. We have no obligation to force care upon capable and mentally competent adults who do not want it. Capable and competent adults have the right to refuse care if they so choose. We do, however, have a duty to make sure that individuals who need care and are incapable of making informed decisions are provided with it. At least until individuals are able to make informed decisions about their care, we should suppose that they wish to survive, develop, and function, and consequently desire the best care available to them. Special oversight is therefore warranted over the care of children and other incapacitated individuals. While mentally competent adults should generally be allowed to care for themselves in whatever manner they choose, their children should be guaranteed a form of care that can be demonstrated to be effective in satisfying their basic biological and developmental needs at adequate levels to survive, develop, and function.

Up to this point, care theory's approach to multicultural practices appears to be not so different from standard liberal approaches. Care theory establishes basic standards for the care of children and other dependents, but then allows parents and other caregivers a good deal

---

[19] Many states in the United States currently have laws to this effect.

of latitude in choosing how to meet these standards (Barry 2001: 203). Care theory begins to depart from standard liberal theories, however, on issues relating to the development of basic capabilities. In *Culture and Equality*, for example, Brian Barry argues that a liberal society ought to provide all children with both a functional education and an education for living well (Barry 2001: 212–25). A functional education aims to develop children's basic reasoning and communication capabilities so that they can function successfully in society. An education for living well aims to develop children's complex capabilities for autonomy, aesthetic appreciation, and other liberal values. Given these goals, Barry suggests that the US Supreme Court ruled wrongly in the case of *Wisconsin* v. *Yoder* when it acknowledged the rights of Amish parents to withdraw their children from school after the age of 14. Even if Amish children have received a functional education by age 14, Barry argues that they have not yet received an education for living well and are unlikely to do so through indoctrination into the Amish way of life (242–4). On similar grounds, he rejects the right of fundamentalist Christian parents to withdraw their children from the public school system in order to enroll them in a Christian school or to educate them at home, since by his estimation doing so often means teaching them the 'mind-destroying' ideas found in fundamentalist Christian textbooks (247–9).

Care theory has more limited educational aims than Barry's liberalism and thus looks differently upon these issues. The aim of education from the perspective of care theory should be more or less what Barry calls a functional education. It should develop students' basic capabilities so that they can function successfully in society. By age 14, most children have developed (or at least should have developed under a good educational system) their basic capabilities to a minimally decent level. Education beyond this point blurs into training for a career, citizenship, or some form of the good life. From the perspective of care theory, the Supreme Court's decision in *Wisconsin* v. *Yoder* therefore seems reasonable. The Amish wished to remove their children from the public education system only after they had presumably developed their basic capabilities in order to train them for a specific form of the good life. If Amish or other (e.g. gypsy) parents wished to deprive their children of a functional education altogether, this would be unacceptable. It also seems acceptable if fundamentalist Christian or other parents wish to send their children to private schools or to educate them at home. The government should stipulate general standards of functioning for these children in areas such as basic reasoning, listening, communicating, reading, writing, and math, and perhaps periodically evaluate students to ensure they are meeting these standards. If, as Barry claims, fundamentalist Christian parents really do provide their children with a mind-destroying education, then government could determine this through evaluations and mandate the return of these children to public education. If these children are adequately developing their innate capabilities, however, then care theory offers no objection to private or home schooling.

Care theory is neutral on other issues of multicultural justice that do not directly affect the ability of individuals to give or receive care, including cultural and language rights, self-determination rights, and so forth. Arguments for or against these group rights must be made for the most part by appealing to values outside of care theory. What matters from the perspective of care theory is that all individuals are able to meet their basic biological and developmental needs. Where cultural marginalization or the lack of self-determination directly impedes some group of individuals from caring for themselves, then care theory supports multicultural rights. Where cultural marginalization or the lack of self-determination rights does not directly impede caring, care theory remains neutral on the question of whether governments should extend rights to various groups. Governments and people must decide these issues for themselves based upon their own visions of the good life. If governments do decide to recognize some sort of group rights, however, care theory further stipulates some limits on group recognition. Specifically, governments have a responsibility to make sure that all individuals within these groups are protected and well cared for (Shachar 2001). Where religious groups are delegated primary control over marriage and divorce laws, for example, governments should concomitantly offer civil marriages and divorces so that individuals can opt out of harmful relationships if necessary. Likewise, if group rules leave some parties without adequate basic resources after a divorce, the government should provide support for these individuals or require the group to do so. In all cases, the government retains residual responsibility for the care of all individuals under its jurisdiction regardless of cultural or religious beliefs.

The general position of care theory on multicultural issues can perhaps be best exemplified by looking at the issue of gay marriage. Gay marriage is a hard case for care theory because it occurs at the intersection between personal caring and conceptions of the good life. On the one hand, gay marriage can be defended within care theory on the grounds that it gives gay partners access to the legal rights, benefits, and responsibilities that support personal caring relationships (Streuning 2002). On the

107

other hand, opponents of gay marriage often portray it as an affront to their religious convictions, their conceptions of marriage, and their understanding of the public good. One way to address this impasse is by distinguishing between the distributional aspects of marriage and its symbolic dimensions.[20] The distributional aspects of marriage include the legal rights and benefits granted to married persons; the symbolic aspects consist of the social recognition bestowed upon legal marriages. Regarding the distributional aspects, it seems important from the perspective of care theory that gay partnerships enjoy the full legal rights, benefits, and responsibilities of heterosexual marriage. Legal entitlements in areas such as medical decision-making, insurance benefits, adoption, and inheritance are important in fostering caring relationships. Regarding the symbolic aspect of gay marriage, however, care theory is neutral. Governments and peoples must decide for themselves whether to grant legal recognition to gay marriage. The arguments for or against symbolic recognition fall outside the scope of care theory and depend upon people's comprehensive moral and religious beliefs. Whether a society grants symbolic recognition to gay marriage would seem to have little effect on the ability of gay partners to care for one another just as long as they enjoy all the legal entitlements of marriage that facilitate caring relationships.

In sum, care theory approaches all questions of multicultural justice by examining their effects on the care of individuals. Care theory generally supports the rights of individuals and groups to give and receive care in culturally diverse ways since personal and local care arrangements generally foster the most attentive, responsive, and respectful forms of caring. Care theory opposes, however, all particular cultural, religious, or other practices that impede the ability of individuals to survive, develop, or function in society. Care theory finally remains neutral toward all practices and traditions that do not directly impact the ability of individuals to give or receive care. Where different groups disagree about whether a particular practice is adequately caring, care theory suggests cross-cultural dialogue oriented around the question of whether the practice effectively satisfies the basic needs of individuals, and whether there are more effective means available for meeting these needs. The ultimate criterion for supporting or opposing any practice under care theory is whether it can be shown to promote or

[20] This approach is loosely based upon Shachar's notion of transformative accommodation (Shachar 2001: 117–45).

impede the ends of individual survival, development, and basic social functioning.

## 2.6. Objections and Responses

The political theory of caring outlined in this chapter is likely to generate a number of objections. Some of these objections may be of an ideological nature and are best addressed through the moral arguments outlined in Chapter 1. Other objections, however, may be of a more practical nature. In this final section, I address some of the more salient of these practical objections.

The most likely objection to a caring political theory is that it is simply too expensive. Subsidized family leaves would cost billions of dollars each year. Childcare subsidies would cost billions more. A country could go bankrupt attempting to provide adequate care for all its people, or have to charge such exorbitant taxes that overall productivity would seriously fall or individuals would be reduced to a bleak social existence.

There are several responses to this first objection. First, no government or people is obligated to support caring policies to the point of bankruptcy. Our duty to care is limited by our resources. If a society is not wealthy enough to care for all individuals, then the government must make use of the limited resources available to it to care for as many individuals as it can. In a similar vein, governments are not obligated to meet the needs of people regardless of the effects on the economy, since this would be counterproductive. One of the central functions of a caring government (as discussed in Chapter 3) is to maintain and promote a stable and prosperous economic and social system where individuals can earn sufficient income to care for themselves and others. Governments would therefore be remiss in their duties if they were to tax people at a rate that seriously undermined economic productivity. The task for government and policy advisors is to find an appropriate tax rate whereby the economy remains stable and prosperous and government can provide care to as many people in need as possible. These issues will be further discussed in Chapter 3. The point here is simply to say that care theory does not endorse support for social programs without regard to their direct or indirect economic costs. A healthy economy is itself a central aim of care theory; the goal of helping others in need must be balanced against this aim.

The core objection nonetheless persists: care policies are too expensive and detrimental to productivity. In response, it may be noted that many European countries already support many of the policies described above with no apparent negative impact on their economic efficiency or productivity (Headey et al. 2000; Rothstein 1998: 23). Indeed, the argument that European-style social programs are incompatible with strong economic performance has been largely discredited (Gornick and Meyers 2003: 283–6). Many of the policies listed above could further be paid for by shifting governmental priorities and raising taxes on average only slightly. In the United States, for example, Helburn and Bergmann estimate that the annual cost of their subsidized childcare program (discussed above) would be about $30 billion above current spending. The US government could pay the costs of this program by cutting agricultural and other corporate subsidies (Helburn and Bergmann 2002: 218–19; Miller 2003: 183–4). A relatively small cut in military spending would probably suffice to pay for a parental leave subsidy. Once established, a national health care system would cost individuals and businesses no more than they are currently spending on medical care. Raising taxes on average by $200 annually per household, distributed fairly according to income, would further yield an additional $21 billion in revenue (Rank 2004: 240). A $400 tax increase would yield $42 billion. The United States and other industrialized countries can thus afford to fund caring programs, and doing so would not bring about the bleak socialist dystopia that opponents of government programs sometimes conjure up. Slight shifts in social priorities and relatively small increases in average taxes would suffice to pay for most of these programs.

In the long term, some of these programs would also likely pay for themselves. The costs of public childcare subsidies, for example, would be largely offset by long-term savings from this program. The better care provided for infants and young children would yield more capable and productive adults who would contribute more to the tax base of society and be less likely to engage in criminal activities or require welfare. As noted above, every dollar spent on enriched preschool programs saves on average between $4 and $6 over the long run in lowered costs for special education, truant officers, welfare benefits, unemployment, court costs, imprisonment, and so forth. Every $1 spent on these programs provides an overall return to society of $17.

It is nonetheless true that a caring political program would be expensive. It would entail increases in government revenues and changes in spending priorities. The main issue, however, is not one of financial

110

feasibility but of morality, and the main moral question is what kind of society we wish to live in. A caring government extends the morality of caring that we all recognize on a personal level to our relations with all individuals throughout society. If this requires an increase in taxes, which it surely will, it nonetheless seems a small price to pay for living in a society in which all individuals have the opportunity to survive, develop, and function at adequate levels.

A second likely objection to a caring political program is that public support for caring will create moral hazards. People may worry, for example, that public support for caring will make it easier for women to have children outside of marriage and thus encourage single-parent families. This objection is usually framed in terms of the child's well-being. Research has found that children of single parent families are more likely to perform poorly in school, drop out of school, have emotional and behavioral problems, get pregnant as teenagers, abuse drugs, and engage in criminal behavior than children from two parent families (Blankenhorn 1995; Galston 1995; Popenoe 1996; Whitehead 1993). The implication would seem to be that our concern for the decent care of children should direct us to deter single parenthood rather than provide any support or encouragement for it. This conclusion, however, does not follow from the research findings. Most of the negative effects associated with single-parent childrearing can be attributed to the lower incomes of single-parent homes, and can be addressed through family subsidies and other policies outlined above (Streuning 2002: xvi, 70–6). The various programs described above would also allow single parents to spend more time with their children and ensure that their children receive adequate care when they are away at work, greatly if not wholly mitigating the negative consequences associated with single parenting. Public support for caring might also serve to promote more two parent homes by relieving couples of some of the strains on time and money that cause so many marriages and partnerships to dissolve.

Some critics might point to another apparent weak spot in this plan: women may choose to have children under a caring government primarily to benefit themselves. Care theory would seem to be especially vulnerable here. It is imperative from the perspective of care theory that all children receive adequate care in the form of sufficient nourishment, clothing, housing, medical care, personal attention, and so forth. Since care theory recommends that governments should attempt to ensure the good care of children primarily by providing support to their parents or primary caregivers, the apparent danger is that blanket support for children and caregiving might provide an incentive for some women to have children as a substitute for engaging in remunerative labor.

In response, it is important first to consider why the prospect of women (or men) collecting benefits for childcare work seems unacceptable to some people. The prejudice seems to stem at least in part from a long liberal tradition that views childcare work as a personal, private, and voluntary responsibility, and not as real work at all. As I argued in Chapter 1, this view is seriously misguided. Children are not like pets, as Nancy Folbre argues, but more like public goods (Folbre 2001: 109–35). We all benefit from the good care that children receive and suffer when they are inadequately cared for. All things considered, society probably has more to gain by supporting mothers (or fathers) in providing good care to their children than it does by forcing them to work minimum wage jobs—especially when quality childcare is not readily available to them.

Some people may nonetheless still be bothered by the possibility that public support for childcare work might encourage women to have children primarily for their own ease or self-interested gain. If women did begin to calculate their pregnancies in this way, there would be reason for concern. Yet few women seem likely to do so. Childbearing and childrearing are difficult and life-altering tasks even with support. When women are offered real opportunities to pursue education, training, and other careers, most choose these other options over childbearing and childrearing (Sen 1999: 217–19). Moreover, welfare benefits do not appear to significantly increase out-of-wedlock births (Albelda et al. 1996: 42–5). In the United States, families on welfare have on average fewer than two children. In European countries where generous child support policies exist, fertility rates are among the lowest in the world. The fear that public support for caring will create significant numbers of career 'welfare moms' thus appears overblown.

There is nevertheless still potential for abuse: it is possible that a few women might have children primarily for the sake of receiving public support. Other individuals might likewise attempt to take advantage of the system of sick leaves, care leaves, or disability benefits for their own ease and comfort. Insofar as these sorts of problems do arise, programs can be designed to minimize the opportunities for abuse. Rather than giving parents direct cash grants to spend on childcare, for example, they might be offered in-kind benefits such as childcare subsidies or vouchers. Certain requirements might similarly be placed on sick leaves, care leaves, and disability benefits—such as authorization by a medical board—to assure that individuals do not misuse them. These options are not ideal, since they introduce punitive elements and bureaucratic requirements into the system of caregiving support. But if abuse of the system is a concern (and as I have tried to show in the case of child benefits, it probably should not be as much of a concern as people have sometimes made it out to be), then remedies can be found to address it. The problem is not so intractable as to undermine the viability of a caring political theory.

Yet another concern about a caring political theory relates to the possibility that public support for caring practices will lead to a weakening of family and social ties (Clement 1996: 97–104). If individuals can count upon the government to subsidize the care of their children or parents, they may make less concerted efforts to care for these individuals on their own. Then family and other social ties may begin to break down. While this critique is usually associated with neoliberal and neoconservative writers, it also finds support in the philosophy of Jurgen Habermas (Habermas 1987: 330–1, 361–4; see also Cohen and Arato 1992: 421–91; Murray 1984; Offe 1988). Habermas argues that if the state aims to support all the needs of its citizens, the natural bonds of family and friendship will become less necessary and natural social relations among people will begin to wither (Rothstein 1998: 24–5). Although there is some reason for concern here, especially with regard to traditional welfare policies, this criticism is misplaced when applied to a caring political theory. As argued above, a caring government will not attempt to displace family and community care but rather to supplement and support it. By providing goods and services to personal caregivers, it makes personal caring more accessible to individuals who might otherwise not be able to provide it adequately on their own (Clement 1996: 100). Far from colonizing civil society, a caring state provides it with a much needed injection of resources so that it can flourish. It enables individuals to care for their children and sick and frail family members by providing them the support and accommodation they need to do so effectively. Moreover, insofar as one takes seriously the duty to care for individuals in need, there really does not seem to be any better alternative to public support for caring activities. If the government does not subsidize caring practices, dependent individuals (e.g. children or elderly parents) may be subjected to poor care simply because their relations lack the financial resources, time, or will to support them. Offering no public support for caregiving, or cutting back the support that already exists, hardly seems likely to solve this problem.

A final practical concern about a caring political theory relates to governmental power (Fineman 2004: 292–307; Roberts 2002: 277–93). Once government becomes involved in supporting caregiving, there is the danger that it will begin to meddle excessively in all matters of human development and health. If we have a duty to assure everyone adequate care, Michael Doyle asks: 'Do we have a moral obligation to act in order to prevent children from perhaps becoming overweight when their parents allow them to consume starchy, fatty foods?' (2006: 111).[21] While child nutrition and health are certainly matters of concern for care theory, a caring government will generally not attempt to regulate these matters in any precise way. Any attempt to regulate too closely parental caring is likely to hinder or diminish the overall quality of caregiving. At the very least, it will make caregivers more subject to bureaucratic rules and hence less attentive and responsive to the particular needs of dependent individuals. It may also unduly impede parents' opportunity to express their identity, practice their culture, or pursue their ideal of the good life in their family and other intimate relations. As long as parents satisfy the basic biological and developmental needs of their children, a caring government will thus leave them alone to care for their children as they see fit—even when aspects of their care may be suboptimal. The goal should be to ensure adequate nutrition and health for all children but not optimal nutrition and health.

Martha Fineman argues in this regard that care theory supports its own sort of privacy policy: 'Thus conceived, privacy would not be a right to separation, secrecy, or seclusion, but rather the right to autonomy or self-determination within the family, even as it is firmly located within a supportive and reciprocal state' (Fineman 2004: 294). Any measure of governmental support and oversight of family care might still seem excessive to some people, but once again, it is not clear that there is any better alternative. Without governmental support and regulation of caring, many individuals will not be able to give or receive adequate care, and many others will be exposed to violence and abuse in their domestic relationships (Fineman 2004: 299). Government may not be a perfect instrument for ensuring the adequate care of all individuals, but without it many people would not be able to give or receive adequate care at all.

---

[21] Doyle raises this question not directly in relation to care theory but in a discussion of Peter Singer's ethical arguments. The question nonetheless is apt for care theory.

## 2.7. Conclusion

Care theory provides a unique definition of the nature and function of a just government. In care theory, government exists primarily to support and accommodate personal caring activities. It does so by serving four main functions: (*a*) it provides security, a clean environment, sanitary water, and other public goods that individuals cannot usually obtain on their own, and guarantees all individuals the basic rights necessary to ensure their safety and the opportunity to care for themselves and others; (*b*) it supports the inevitable dependencies of human life including childhood, sickness and injury, and disability and old age; (*c*) it offers temporary support and subsidies to capable individuals who for some good reason cannot adequately care for themselves and their dependents; and (*d*) it guarantees people a responsive government. A caring government departs from traditional welfare policies by focusing on proactive programs aimed at lending support to personal caring activities. It further offers a unique approach to issues of multicultural justice that measures the morality of different practices and customs according to their effectiveness in helping individuals to satisfy their biological and developmental needs. While a caring government, like other forms of government, comes with certain costs and problems, none of these potential drawbacks are serious enough to render a caring political program unfeasible.

This chapter has focused on the political institutions and policies of a caring society. In Chapter 3, I supplement this argument by outlining care theory's approach to economic justice. The political institutions and policies outlined in this chapter are not sufficient by themselves to support and accommodate personal caring activities. Care theory must also be brought to bear on the economic institutions and policies of society.

# 3

# Care Theory and Economic Justice

Contemporary political and economic theorists have outlined a variety of approaches to economic justice, including libertarian, welfare liberal, market socialist, communist, and other perspectives.[1] Few of these theorists, however, have given much attention to the place of caring practices in a just economy.[2] Rather, most mainstream theorists have taken caring practices for granted or treated them as private and unproductive activities, and hence left them out of their accounts of economic justice.

In recent years, feminist theorists have begun to challenge these views and develop an alternative account of economic justice organized around the practice of caring (Bubeck 1995; Donath 2000; Folbre 2001; Gardiner 1997; Held 1993, 2002, 2006; Jochimsen 2003; Nelson 1993; Schwarzenbach 1987, 1996). These theorists argue that caring practices deserve a central place in any theory of economic justice because they are a necessary precondition for economic activity. Caring practices sustain and replenish workers so that they can engage in commodity production, prepare children to enter into the labor force, and help temporarily sick and disabled individuals to return to work. As such, traditional distinctions between the economy and home, 'productive labor' and 'unproductive' caring practices, make little sense. Most people further work primarily for the sake of caring for themselves and their loved ones. In this respect, the goals of caring may be said to provide a central normative justification

---

[1] See, e.g., Friedman (1982), Miller (1989), Nozick (1974), Ollman (1979, 1998), Rawls (1999), Roemer (1996), and Schweickart (1993, 2002).

[2] In outlining his account of market socialism, Schweickart does note, as an aside, that a market socialist economy would include provisions for childcare, health care, and other care services (2002: 71–6). However, he provides very little discussion of these policies, and instead devotes the vast majority of his book to describing and defending his account of market socialist instititutions.

for most forms of work.[3] Any economic system that fails to support and accommodate the ability of individuals to care for themselves and their loved ones subverts one of the primary reasons most people have for supporting and complying with it.

While feminist theorists have outlined the basic tenets of a caring theory of economic justice, they have only partially described its substantive principles and policies. In this chapter, I build upon their arguments in order to elaborate more fully the economic institutions and policies of a caring society. In Section 3.1, I outline the basic concepts and moral orientation of a caring economic theory. In Section 3.2, I discuss Virginia Held's and Nancy Folbre's important accounts of care theory and economic justice. While Held and Folbre identify some of the central goals and policies of a caring economic theory, both focus primarily on personal care activities and direct care services within the economy. Neither considers in any detail how economic institutions and policies can be organized more generally to facilitate the ability of individuals to care for themselves and others. Section 3.3 takes up this subject by exploring the economic system (communism, market socialism, market capitalism, etc.) most conducive to supporting and accommodating caring activities. In Section 3.4, I formulate six general principles for establishing and maintaining a caring economic system, and describe in some detail the economic policies following from them. In Section 3.5, I briefly explore the viability of a caring economic system in context of economic globalization.

Care theory offers a new approach to economic justice. It departs from liberal, Marxist, and other economic theories by reorienting economic institutions and policymaking around a set of concerns that have generally not found a place within accounts of economic justice. The central goals of a caring economy may be summarized as: ensuring that everyone has access to the economic resources necessary to care for themselves and their dependents, ensuring that economic activities do not unduly interfere with the ability of individuals to care for themselves and their dependents, and supporting and subsidizing direct service care and personal caring activities as necessary. Liberal, Marxist, and other normative economic theories have generally set their sights on grander and more abstract goals such as fostering free and equal exchange or abolishing exploitative labor practices. Care theory endeavors more basically

---

[3] As I argue below, this does not mean that most forms of productive work are caring, but only that most forms of productive work exist most fundamentally for the sake of supporting caring practices.

to organize economic institutions and policies so that they provide all individuals with the real opportunity to care adequately for themselves, their loved ones, and human beings in general.

## 3.1. A Caring Approach to Economic Justice

Care theory's approach to economic justice can be traced back in part to the domestic labor dispute of the 1960s and 1970s. In the domestic labor dispute, Marxist feminists attempted to link women's domestic labor to capitalist exploitation in order to show that feminist concerns about unpaid housework were not reactionary or bourgeois but central to the revolutionary class struggle itself (Bubeck 1995: 17–83; Gardiner 1997: 56–99). Mariarosa Dalla Costa and Selma James's *The Power of Women and the Subversion of the Community* represents one of the most important and influential statements of this position.[4] While Marx argued that domestic labor was a form of unproductive labor that falls 'outside the process of producing commodities', Dalla Costa and James countered that women's domestic labor is actually the 'very pillar of the capitalist organization of work' (Dalla Costa and James 1975: 35; Marx 1976: 1004; Smith 1978: 211–12). Women's domestic labor frees men to leave home and enter into the labor force, and replenishes their labor power when they return home (34). It likewise prepares children for their roles as the next generation of workers. Far from being valueless or unproductive, then, domestic labor is 'essential to the production of surplus value' and 'productive in the Marxian sense' (33, 53 n. 12). It lies behind commodity production and makes the generation of surplus value possible. The failure to appreciate this point, according to Dalla Costa and James, has impeded the class struggle and helped to prop up the capitalist system:

If we fail to grasp completely that precisely this family [where women perform domestic labor] is the very pillar of the capitalist organization of work, if we make the mistake of regarding it only as a superstructure, dependent for change only on the stages of the struggle in the factories, then we will be moving in a limping revolution that will always perpetuate and aggravate *a basic contradiction in the class struggle, and a contradiction which is functional to capitalist development*. We would,

---

[4] There is some confusion about the authorship of this work. Bubeck identifies Dalla Costa as the sole author of the essay *Women and the Subversion of Community* (Bubeck 1995: 52). Yet the Foreward and Publishers' Note identify both James and Dalla Costa as the authors (1975: 4).

in other words, be perpetuating the error of considering ourselves as producers of use values only, of considering housewives external to the working class. As long as housewives are considered external to the class, the class struggle at every moment and any point is impeded, frustrated, and unable to find full scope for its action. (35)

Stated more succinctly, women's liberation is essential to the class struggle. Calls for wages for housework and the like are not reactionary or bourgeois demands but part of the revolutionary fight itself.

Despite the seeming plausibility of Dalla Costa and James's thesis, orthodox Marxist theorists roundly criticized their argument as confused and lacking in rigor. Wally Seccombe argued, for example, that Dalla Costa and James misapplied the Marxist category of productive labor to domestic labor.[5] 'Nowhere do they maintain that the housewife works in direct relation with capital and yet they appear unaware that the directness of this relation is the central criterion of productive labour' (Seccombe 1974: 11 n. 16). Dalla Costa and James similarly overextended the Marxist concept of exploitation: 'The housewife, in Marxist terms, is unexploited because surplus value is not extracted from her labour. To say this is not as James and Dalla Costa imply, to be soft on women's oppression. The housewife is intensely *oppressed* within the nuclear family under capitalism, but she is not *exploited*' (Seccombe 1974: 11 n. 16). Paul Smith further noted that Dalla Costa and James fail to recognize important differences between commodity production and domestic labor (1978). While commodity production creates goods that can be exchanged and consumed, domestic labor aims primarily at sustaining and developing human beings. Likewise, while wage laborers will chase high wages from one job to another, women will continue to perform domestic labor regardless of wages and even when there is 'relative overproduction of its particular good' (Smith 1978: 204, 206). As such, Smith concluded that domestic labor does not and cannot form part of the capitalist mode of production. It is not a form of abstract and productive labor, and consequently, does not form part of the class struggle against capitalism.

While the domestic labor debate was ultimately something of a 'dead end' from a feminist standpoint, it does help to highlight the limits of Marxism from a caring perspective (Bubeck 1995: 8; Gardiner 1997: 5). Marxism aims primarily at ending exploitative and alienating production and achieving worker autonomy over the products and processes of their

---

[5] Seccombe's name is misspelled on the first page of his article 'The Housewife and Her Labour under Capitalism' in the *New Left Review*. The correct spelling is Seccombe, not Secombe.

labor. Care theory aims more basically at helping individuals to survive, develop, and achieve basic social functioning. Marxists have traditionally not been very interested in care because it does not easily fit into their conception of exploited productive labor. Just as care theory cannot, then, look to liberal theory to articulate and support its concerns about political justice, neither can it look to Marxism to articulate its concerns about economic justice.

Care theory instead offers a new orientation to economic justice. The basic goal of a caring economic theory is to organize economic activities to support and accommodate caring practices. Caring practices include everything we do directly to help human beings: (*a*) to meet their basic needs for food, sanitary water, shelter, clothing, basic medical care, a clean environment, rest, and protection; (*b*) to develop or sustain their basic capabilities for sensation, mobility, emotion, reason, speech, imagination, affiliation, reading, writing, and numeracy; and (*c*) to live as much as possible free from unwanted or unnecessary pain and suffering. Caring, so defined, overlaps in part with the category of domestic labor, but is different from it. On the one hand, caring practices are broader than domestic labor practices because they include the medical fields, teaching, elder care, and other caring services that regularly take place outside the home. On the other hand, caring practices are narrower than domestic labor activities because they encompass only those parts of domestic labor that directly contribute to human survival, development, and functioning. While some measure of cooking, cleaning, and other domestic chores is certainly necessary for supporting the survival and healthy development of human beings, not all domestic chores directly contribute to these ends. The practical significance of this distinction is that care theory does not support the broad feminist demand for wages for housework, but favors only subsidies for those portions of housework associated directly with caring for dependent individuals.

Since most forms of productive work ultimately contribute to the satisfaction of human biological and developmental needs, this definition of caring might seem overly broad. As argued in Chapter 1, caring practices may nonetheless be distinguished from most forms of productive work by their direct or proximate aims. Caring practices include only those activities that aim *directly* at helping individuals to satisfy their needs. Examples include feeding, clothing, sheltering, healing, protecting, rehabilitating, teaching, and soothing, as well as supplying provisions for these activities. Most productive economic activities, by contrast, aim directly at growing, harvesting, extracting, manufacturing, shipping, or selling commodities.

The proximate aim of a tomato farmer is to grow and harvest tomatoes. The proximate aim of a trucker is to transport the tomatoes to a canning factory. The proximate aim of a factory worker is to put the tomatoes in a can. Even though all these activities ultimately aim to satisfy needs and support caring activities, they all have more immediate or proximate aims and therefore are not themselves caring. All of them can be successfully completed without directly helping individuals to satisfy their biological or developmental needs. Even the chef in a restaurant has proximate aims other than those of meeting the needs of individuals. His or her direct goal is to make and sell a meal, at which point his or her work has been successfully completed. The customer who buys the meal may, or may not, put the meal to caring uses. (He or she may, after all, also dump it into his or her lover's lap.) By contrast, a parent successfully completes his or her work of cooking for a child only when the child actually ingests nourishing food. Preparing a meal for a child is therefore caring in a way that cooking a meal in a restaurant usually is not.[6] If the chef were to volunteer his or her services to help feed the homeless, of course, then his or her actions would in this case be caring.

The distinction between commodity production and caring practices should not be mistaken for a distinction between paid and unpaid work. Teachers, doctors, nurses, childcare providers, and others all earn wages by caring for others. The fact that their caregiving is paid does not render it uncaring. Indeed, paid caring is often superior to unpaid caring. A doctor or child psychologist may be better able to identify and address a child's needs for medical care or emotional support than his or her parents are capable of doing (Folbre and Nelson 2000: 135). The distinction between caring practices and commodity labor depends not on whether the work is paid but on the direct aims of the activity itself. Most of the work of teachers, doctors, nurses, and childcare providers aims directly at satisfying the biological and developmental needs of individuals.[7] When one

---

[6] Sibyl Schwarzenbach makes a similar distinction between craft labor and caring activities: 'Whereas the immediate aim or purpose of the art, say, of shoe-making (as Socrates argued) is to produce good shoes (whether or not this is done for money), it is clear that the aim of child-care is to encourage the healthy development of the child. The ultimate "for the sake of which" the activity is performed is to produce a mature, functioning adult. Thus, where craft labor may be said to aim *in*directly at the satisfaction of human needs ("good" shoes after all are those which produce "happy feet"), female labor aims *directly* at it' (1987: 154). My account of caring practices is nonetheless distinct from Schwarzenbach's in that she defines all craft labor as noncaring, whereas in my framework, the production of goods can be caring (e.g. cooking a meal, knitting a sweater) insofar as it is done for the direct aim of satisfying human needs.

[7] An exception here would be doctors who perform unnecessary cosmetic surgery.

purchases their services, one pays for their direct care (a use value) rather than a discrete commodity that may or may not be used for caring purposes. Commodity production, by contrast, aims at the manufacture and distribution of goods and always requires the intervention of a caregiver to put its products to caring uses.

Our obligation to organize our economic institutions to support caring practices follows from our dependency upon other human beings. We have all made claims upon other human beings for care, and in the process, implicitly committed ourselves to the general moral principle that capable human beings ought to care for other human beings in need when they are able to do so. Since we can personally care for only a few individuals by ourselves, our obligation to care for others further directs us to establish collective caring institutions that can aid and support individuals beyond our reach or means. In economic matters, this means organizing, supporting, and complying with economic institutions and policies that support the ability of individuals to care for themselves and their dependents. Any economic arrangements that fail to meet these goals are contrary to the moral duties arising from our dependent nature.

Economic institutions and policies that fail to support human care can also be said to contradict their own implicit moral goals. As noted above, caring practices sustain and reproduce the productive economy. Any economic system that fails to support and accommodate caring practices therefore corrodes the foundations of its own existence. Of course, caring practices also depend upon commodity production. Without the resources and raw materials of commodity production, individuals would not be able to care for themselves or others. Caring and commodity production thus must be balanced. Yet, while commodity production and caring practices can be said to represent two independent and interdependent material bases of human life, caring practices may be said to have some moral priority over commodity production. Although people may engage in commodity production for a variety of reasons—to earn money, grow wealthy, become powerful, assert their identity, or simply because they enjoy it—we all necessarily work or depend upon the work of others in order to care for ourselves and our dependents. Productive work provides us with the food, raw materials, wages, and other economic goods that we can use to satisfy our basic needs and the needs of our dependents. As such, commodity production may be said to be most fundamentally oriented around the moral goal of supporting human caring. This does not mean, of course, that all commodity production is caring.

The proximate aims of commodity production are usually different from the aims of caring practices and have distinctive aims and virtues that guide them. Most forms of commodity production nonetheless exist most basically for the sake of supporting caring practices. It therefore makes sense from a moral standpoint to subordinate commodity production at least in part to the moral aims of caring.

In *The Great Transformation* ([1944] 2001), Karl Polanyi provides a historical and theoretical approach to economic justice that generally supports this understanding of the moral relationship between caring practices and commodity production, and also helps to contextualize existing relations between caring practices and commodity production in most industrial societies. Polanyi argues that nearly all societies throughout history have embedded economic production within a set of social goals (45–58). These social goals have included religious beliefs, cultural practices, and customary and status systems, but have focused most fundamentally on addressing the needs of human beings. In fact, Polanyi argues that one of the primary functions of custom, law, magic, and religion in most societies has been to induce individuals to direct their economic activities toward cooperative ends (57).

The communal and caring organization of economic activities is not accidental or a primitive feature of social organization, according to Polanyi, but follows from the social nature of human beings and our necessary dependency on others. 'For if one conclusion stands out more clearly than another from the recent study of early societies, it is the changelessness of man as a social being. His natural endowments reappear with a remarkable constancy in societies of all times and places; and the necessary preconditions of the survival of human society appear to be immutably the same' (48). Because human beings necessarily depend upon one another to meet our survival and developmental needs, nearly all societies have historically organized productive economic activities to help all their members meet their needs:

The outstanding discovery of recent historical and anthropological research is that man's economy, as a rule, is submerged in his social relationships. He does not act so as to safeguard his individual interest in the possession of material goods; he acts so as to safeguard his social standing, his social claims, his social assets. He values material goods only in so far as they serve this end. ... The explanation, in terms of survival, is simple. Take the case of a tribal society. The individual's economic interest is rarely paramount, for the community keeps all its members from starving unless it is itself borne down by catastrophe, in which case interests are again threatened collectively, not individually. (48)

Polanyi goes on to argue that the moral goal of social caring has provided the central organizing principle of economic production for nearly all societies until recent times. 'The principle of freedom from want was equally acknowledged in the Indian village community and, we might add, under almost every and any type of social organization up to about the beginning of sixteenth-century Europe' (171–2).

The great transformation in economic organization occurred in the West during the nineteenth century, though there were presentiments of this transformation as early as the sixteenth century. Governments took steps to free up land, labor, and money for use in capitalist markets (59–70, 141–209). Previously regulated markets were deregulated and transformed into 'self-regulating markets' without government controls. Individuals were cast out of traditional work and livelihoods to make their own way in new employment markets. Traditional social supports were abolished, and market forces were allowed to overtake society. In this new social framework, 'instead of economy being embedded in social relations, social relations are embedded in the economic system' (60). Released from social goals, individuals could now accumulate tremendous wealth without regard for others, and individuals who did not or could not succeed in the free market were left mainly to their own devices to survive.

The natural tendency of these developments, according to Polanyi, was to destroy human life and society. 'Our idea is that the idea of a self-adjusting market implied a stark utopia. Such an institution could not exist for any length of time without annihilating the human and natural substance of society; it would have physically destroyed man and transformed his surroundings into a wilderness' (3). Because the self-adjusting or unregulated free market was so disruptive of basic social institutions and practices, it inevitably gave rise to a countermovement among people to protect themselves and society (79–80). Marx saw the countermovement as rooted in class interests, but Polanyi argues that it actually had a broader social base (158–70). Since the free market ideology threatened the social institutions and practices necessary to sustain human life and society, individuals belonging to various economic strata joined forces to resist it (162). The most visible expressions of this countermovement included the enactment of protectionist policies and trade tariffs designed to buffer individuals and national industries from free trade, the growth of labor unions and business cartels, and the intensification of nationalist sentiments. The struggle between the two movements of the period—on the one side, the push for greater economic liberalism and, on the other side, the demand for more economic and social protections—eventually brought the entire system to the point of collapse, and gave rise to the authoritarian fascist and communist movements of the 1920s and 1930s.

Polanyi believed that the misguided dream of a self-regulating free-market society had just about been exhausted by the close of World War II, and he looked forward to a postwar world that would restore the priority of social goals over market relations (249–58). The postwar years did in fact bring a new commitment to social aims over economic gains. Keynesian ideas dominated economic policy in most Western countries through the 1960s (Block 2001: xx). The cold war likewise ensured that political considerations predominated over strictly economic ones. By the 1980s, however, the market system was resurgent, and following the collapse of the Soviet Union, Western governments and international organizations forcefully pressed to reestablish self-regulating markets throughout the world (Beneria 2003: 65–74). The ascendancy of the market today mirrors in many ways the dominance of free-market ideals during the late nineteenth and early twentieth centuries. Under neoliberal adjustment plans, countries are being pressured to loosen controls over labor and capital and cut back their social support programs to allow for the full ascendancy of the free market. The recent resurgence of nationalism and socialism in several Latin American countries may be seen as one contemporary countermovement against these policies.

Care theory aims to re-embed the economy within society by reorienting economic processes around the goal of supporting caring practices. It attempts to restore the balance between caring and commodity production that has marked most societies throughout history, and was abandoned in capitalist countries only over the past couple of centuries. More generally, it aims to realign commodity production with its implicit normative purpose of supporting and promoting human survival, development, and basic social functioning. Care theory nonetheless does not attempt to entirely submerge commodity production to the goals of caring. As argued in Chapters 1 and 2, care theory is an incomplete theory of justice. It identifies a set of basic moral goals for economic organization but does not attempt to define the all-encompassing ends of economic activity. Human beings might legitimately choose to organize their economic institutions and policies to promote some vision of the good life above and beyond caregiving, such as individual freedom, worker autonomy, or religious virtue. Any of these visions of the economic good life is acceptable to care theory just as long as it does not impede the ability of individuals to give and receive decent care. Care theory aims only to tether commodity production to the fundamental normative purpose of supporting and accommodating caring practices. An economic order that fails in this regard violates the basic moral principles that follow from human beings' dependent nature and are necessary for producing and reproducing human life and society.

## 3.2. Economic Justice and Direct Care Services

Feminist theorists have outlined a number of strategies for incorporating caring practices into accounts of economic justice (Meagher and Nelson 2004). Some have called for the inclusion of caring labor in the measure of gross domestic product both to recognize caregivers' contributions to economic productivity and to redefine conceptions of prosperity (Folbre 2001: 53–80; Waring 1988). Others have called more generally for a new approach to economics focusing 'on the provisioning of human life, that is, on the commodities and processes necessary to human survival' (Nelson 1993: 32; see also Donath 2000). The most complete and detailed accounts of a specifically caring approach to economic justice, however, have been outlined by Virginia Held and Nancy Folbre.[8] Both suggest strategies for reforming economic institutions and policies so that they better support direct care services within the economy, including education, health care, and childcare.

In *Feminist Morality*, Held explores 'what society would look like, for both descriptive and prescriptive purposes, if we replaced the paradigm of economic man with the paradigm of mother and child' (Held 1993: 195). Since Held develops her account of care theory from the perspective of the mother–child relation, her argument has some of the limitations of the maternalist approaches discussed in Chapter 1. Nonetheless, much of her analysis is still useful in highlighting the limitations of liberal market approaches in supporting caring activities. Even though caring relationships are not always as emotionally charged as mother–child relationships, many have at least some of the general characteristics of mother–child relationships that she describes.

Held first notes that caring relations are distinct from market relations because they are usually less voluntary and consensual (Held 1993:

---

[8] Sibyl Schwarzenbach (1987), Joan Tronto (1993), Diemut Elisabet Bubeck (1995), Eva Kittay (1999), and Joan Williams (2001) have also provided partial accounts of economic justice from a care perspective. Their ideas will be discussed below in more fully developing a caring economic theory.

204–5). Mothers and children are bound together by affection, solicitude, and responsibility rather than self-interest and free choice, and neither mother nor child gets to choose the other in the way a customer might choose which products to buy. Many other caring relationships share some of these qualities. Elderly, sick, disabled, and other dependent individuals often have limited choices over who will care for them, and both personal and professional caregivers often perform their work at least in part out of a sense of obligation to others. Market relations are also usually driven by self-interest, whereas 'the emotional satisfaction of a person engaged in mothering arises from the well-being and happiness of another human being and from the health of the relation between two persons, not the gain that results from an egoistic bargain' (205). A similar point can be made about other caring practices. The central aim in caring for others is to foster their survival, development, and functioning. Self-interested gain is usually (or at least ideally) secondary. Power also functions very differently in market and caring relationships. In the capitalist market, unequal power relations usually mean that the more powerful party can manipulate the weaker party into accepting unfair terms of exchange. By contrast, in caring relations, the ostensibly more powerful party—the caregiver—serves the dependent person and is usually most beholden to this person when he or she is the most vulnerable, such as in infancy and illness (209).

Held highlights these and other differences between market and caring relations not in order to impugn market relations, but to demonstrate their limited applicability. Even though caring relations are fundamental to individual survival and social reproduction, the model of 'contractual relations between self-interested or mutually disinterested individuals' has often been taken as paradigmatic for all human relations (Held 1993: 194, 1995: 131). Held suggests that we should reverse this perspective so that the practices of caring are placed at 'the "heart" or "foundation" or "core" of society', and market relations are put in their (limited) place (Held 1993: 72):

When we explore the implications of these speculations we may come to realize that instead of seeing the family as an anomalous island in a sea of rational contracts making up economic and political and social life, perhaps it is instead economic man who belongs on a relatively small island surrounded by social ties of a less hostile, cold, and precarious kind. (214)

By Held's account, self-interested and voluntary exchange makes up only a small part of most people's lives. Since caring practices, by contrast, are essential for individual functioning and social reproduction, she suggests that they should be recognized and supported as unique and important activities apart from market ideals.

Held ultimately argues that no one set of goals or values should govern all activities: each domain should be guided by the goals and values most appropriate to it (1993: 195, 218).[9] Commodity production and exchange should be guided by utilitarian values that allow individuals to maximize their preference satisfaction (1993: 218–19, 224). By contrast, childcare, education, health care, and other practices where the production and reproduction of human life is the goal should be governed by the aims and virtues of caring.

We can recognize domains in which the individual pursuit of self-interest and the maximization of individual satisfactions are morally permissible, but we can also see how this framework and these values should not be extended to the whole of human activity and society. In practices such as those involved in education, child care, health care, culture, and protecting the environment, market norms limited only by rights should not prevail, even if the market is fair and efficient, because markets are unable to express and promote many values important to these practices, such as mutually shared caring concern. (2006: 120)

According to Held, caring aims and virtues cannot find adequate expression through free market exchange and competition. When caring activities are subordinated to the goals of moneymaking and self-interested gain, they are invariably distorted and constrained. In order to protect the domains of caring from market forces, Held thus suggests that most education, childcare, health care, cultural institutions, and environmental activities should be taken out of the market and publicly supported (2006: 122). By her account, this is the only way to ensure that the aims and values of caring will prevail in these domains rather than self-interest and the profit motive. As she writes of education: 'Once an educational institution or activity has been taken over by the market, anything other than economic gain cannot be its highest priority, since a corporation's responsibility to its shareholders requires it to try to maximize economic gain' (2006: 115). Held is nonetheless careful to point out that insulating the caring domains from market pressures does not mean eliminating all competition, experimentation, and efficiency from them (2006: 121–2). Competition, experimentation, and efficiency should still be promoted in schools, hospitals, and other caring institutions, but they should be used to augment the goals of caring rather than constrain them. When

[9] Held further develops this argument for domains of justice in *Rights and Goods* (1984).

decisions about good caring are driven by concerns about economic gain, the result is usually a diminution in the quality of care.

In *The Invisible Heart* (2001) and numerous articles, Nancy Folbre further elaborates on these themes, describing the various ways in which the 'invisible hand' of market capitalism devalues and disrupts 'the invisible heart' of caring. Like Held, Folbre emphasizes the important contributions that caring practices make to human well-being and the functioning of the market society.

Parents who raise happy, healthy, and successful children create an especially important public good. Children themselves are not the only beneficiaries. Employers profit from access to productive workers. The elderly benefit from Social Security taxes paid by the younger generation.... Fellow citizens gain from having productive and law-abiding neighbors. These are all examples of positive spillovers and side effects that economists often call 'positive externalities' because they are external to the actual decision to provide care. (2001: 50)

Capitalist markets nonetheless tend to penalize individuals who engage in caring activities, thus undermining the very practices they depend upon for their existence (Folbre 2001: 22–52). Individuals (usually women) who take time out from the paid labor market to care for children or sick or elderly relations not only may receive no monetary compensation for their care work, but also tend to earn less income over time because they miss out on promotions and training opportunities or are viewed as unreliable employees. Similarly, people who work in the caring professions in the United States, including teachers, counselors, childcare workers, social workers, and nurses, are paid on average 5 to 6 percent less than people in other occupations after controlling for education and employment experience (England, Budig, and Folbre 2002). The pay penalty is especially hard on female childcare workers who suffer a 41 percent penalty for performing this form of care work. Folbre and her colleagues hypothesize several explanations for the low pay of care work. 'It often serves clients with little or no ability to pay, it involves a function culturally associated with women, and thus devalued, and care work has not been able to take advantage of the productivity per worker increases from capitalist investment to the extent that other work has' (England, Budig, and Folbre 2002: 468–9). This last point is especially important. Because care work is inherently labor intensive, it tends to be expensive and not very profitable. There is little that capitalist entrepreneurs can do to increase the productivity of care work aside from increasing the workload of caregivers and paying them as little as possible, both of which tend to reduce the quality of caregiving. Folbre further notes a fourth reason why many forms of care work may be poorly paid: 'Care providers are not in a very good position to bargain for more resources, because such bargaining puts the people they are caring for at risk' (Folbre 2001: 40). In many cases, care workers may sacrifice increases in their own wages or free time or endure poor working conditions so that they can continue caring for clients whom they feel an obligation to serve.

Folbre further documents the corrosive effects that market competition and low wages have on direct care services in the United States. The for-profit systems of elder care and childcare generally translate into under-staffing, high burn-out rates among workers, and less personal contact between care professionals and their clients (Folbre 2001: 57–64; see also Folbre and Nelson 2000). Close to 40 percent of nursing homes in the United States have repeatedly failed to pass the most basic health and safety inspections, and turnover rates among nursing home aides amount to almost 100 percent within the first three months of employment (Folbre 2001: 61, 2006: 21). Many childcare facilities are likewise over-crowded, staffed by unqualified workers, have high employee turnover rates, and fail to meet basic quality standards (Helburn and Bergmann 2002: 87–122). Similar dynamics prevail in the for-profit health care sys-tem. Competition among health care providers creates incentives to min-imize hospital stays, limit the clinical options of doctors, and substitute unlicensed 'care technicians' for registered nurses. Providers succeed in this system not so much by increasing the quality of care but by avoiding unhealthy patients and reducing services. 'This creates the paradox of a health care system based on avoiding the sick' (Physicians' Working Group 2003: 798). Since improving care in any of these fields would almost surely diminish their profitability, improvements are unlikely to come without some sort of government intervention. The unique aims and virtues of caring mean that caring practices are unlikely ever to be very well supported or compensated by unregulated market competition.

Folbre proposes a slightly different solution from Held for addressing the inadequacies of the market in supporting caring practices. Whereas Held suggests that we should remove direct care services entirely from the market and provide them with public support, Folbre argues that at least some direct care services might successfully exist within the market given adequate government support and regulation (Folbre 2006; Folbre and Nelson 2000). In discussing childcare, for example, she outlines two possible alternatives (Folbre 2000). The first, based on the French model, would look to the government to establish public early education and childcare centers for all young children. The second, market-based strategy would provide childcare subsidies or vouchers to all parents that they could use to purchase childcare from private providers subject to government regulations.[10] Folbre similarly suggests that some of the problems in the medical and elder care industries might be rectified by stronger and more extensive regulatory standards such as minimum nurse-to-patient staffing ratios (Folbre 2006: 24). In other areas, however, Folbre suggests solutions more in line with Held's approach. She argues, for instance, that more public education funding is generally preferable to privatized approaches to educational reform, though she does hold out the possibility that a voucher program might be acceptable 'if equality of educational access were guaranteed and quality standards were enforced at both private and public schools' (Folbre 2001: 152). She more generally argues that the government ought to provide public support for various forms of personal caregiving, such as offering guaranteed paid leaves for new mothers and fathers, family tax credits, and a decent minimal income for poor families with children (Folbre 2001: 109–35, 225–32).

Despite their differences, both Held and Folbre agree that caring activities should be protected against the corrosive effects of market competition. The question of whose approach is better is ultimately an empirical one that may admit to more than one answer. Held's claim that commodification is always deleterious to caring is probably overstated. It rests on an exaggerated characterization of the market as inherently cold, mechanical, and heartless (Nelson 2006). Given adequate government subsidies and regulations, there would seem no reason why market processes might not be able to support and promote at least some caring practices. Nonetheless, Held may be correct to say that at least some direct care services—say, education and health care—can only be effectively provided outside the market. Different types of direct care services may in fact be best served by different public–private arrangements. Childcare, for example, might work well through a voucher program, but education might not. Julie Nelson writes in this regard:

The real issue, then, is not about 'the reach of the market' (to quote [Held 2002: 32]) but about the reach of perverse values and uncaring, disrespectful relationships. Our focus could more helpfully shift to a more specific concern about values, motivations, and responsibilities in all sorts of organizations and social institutions. Social science has its work cut out for it: after a priori blanket prejudgments

---

[10] Folbre does express a preference for a more universal, 'less market-based approach' to childcare, but notes some advantages of the voucher system (2000).

about the bliss-inducing (neoliberal theory) or misery-inducing (critical theory) inexorable effects of markets are set aside, there remains the crucial and fascinating job of investigating the specific sorts of processes and social arrangements that are most likely to lead to positive, humane outcomes. (Nelson 2006: 1071)

Care theory remains flexible when it comes to defining the best means for delivering care, favoring experimentation and innovation to determine the most suitable care arrangements in different social contexts. What is nonetheless clear from Held's and Folbre's analyses is that direct care services need to be sheltered at least in part from market competition in order to allow their aims and virtues to find full expression.

While Held and Folbre describe a core part of a caring economic program, their theories are ultimately limited. Held argues that the caring domains should be removed and protected from the greater economy, but says very little about the institutions and policies of the greater economy. Folbre proposes a number of policies to support personal care activities and direct care services, but likewise makes only passing reference to general economic institutions and policies. Held's and Folbre's narrow focus on direct care services and personal caring activities is certainly understandable given that a caring economic order will be centrally concerned with supporting these practices. However, some attention must also be given to larger questions of institutional and policy design. Economic institutions and policies determine in large part the production and distribution of economic goods, which in turn largely determines the resources that individuals have available to them to care for themselves and others. If individuals do not have access to jobs and wages, they are unlikely to be able to support adequate care for themselves or their dependents. If they must work overly long hours or under harsh conditions, they may likewise not have the time and energy to care adequately for themselves or their dependents. If, then, we are concerned to organize the economy to support and accommodate caring practices, we must look beyond public support for direct care services in order to consider how we can best arrange economic institutions and policies so that they provide all individuals with real opportunities to obtain the resources and have the time and energy to care adequately for themselves and others. That is, we must think more broadly about whether the productive economy supports what Julie Nelson calls 'the provisioning of human life' (1993: 32). Unless the economy at large is supportive of personal caring practices, many people will not be able to care for themselves and others despite public support for direct care services. Our duty to care for others thus ultimately directs us to consider the general economic institutions and policies that are most conducive to supporting and accommodating adequate care for all individuals.

## 3.3. The General Institutions of a Caring Economy

In developing this broader account of a caring economic theory, the first question to be addressed is whether any one form of macroeconomic system is best suited to supporting caring practices. Some care theorists have argued, for example, that care theory necessarily involves a socialist form of economic organization. Joan Tronto writes that care theory 'is probably ultimately anti-capitalistic because it posits meeting needs of care, rather than the pursuit of profit, as the highest social goal' (Tronto 1993: 175). Sibyl Schwarzenbach argues on similar grounds that caring relations are more compatible with socialist ownership and a gift economy than with private property and market competition (Schwarzenbach 1987). Other feminist economists have similarly juxtaposed care 'to the assumed inherent injustices of capitalist employer–worker relations and the assumed heartlessness of profit-making enterprise' and at least implied that socialism or communism is better suited than market capitalism for supporting caring practices (Nelson 2006).

While neither Tronto nor Schwarzenbach develops the case for socialism from a caring perspective in any detail, their claims seem plausible enough. Capitalist ownership and market competition would appear to be incompatible with the aims and virtues of caring in at least four ways. First, capitalist production and exchange is driven by profits and consumer demand rather than human needs. In an effort to maximize profits, capitalist enterprises produce goods exclusively for individuals with money to spend rather than attending to individual needs. There is thus no necessary connection between capitalist production and the satisfaction of human needs. Rather, capitalist economies are likely to produce a preponderance of luxury items for wealthy consumers and an undersupply of basic goods that might improve the lives of poor individuals. Housebuilders, for example, may attempt to maximize profits by building many expensive mansions despite a shortage of low-income housing for the poor. If individuals do not have money to spend, capitalist producers will generally not respond to their needs.

Second, as Held and Folbre argue, capitalist economies also tend to undermine caring practices. Businesses often see little reason to support and accommodate personal caring practices since they can generally reap the benefits of personal caring (e.g. by hiring already grown and capable workers) without having to pay for it. They likewise have little incentive to provide for elderly or disabled individuals who may never return to work or engage in productive labor. Care workers, in turn, tend to be underpaid and undervalued by capitalist markets, and capitalist competition drives private care providers to maximize the quantity of care they can supply at the lowest possible cost, thus generally lowering the quality of care they provide to individuals.

Ruth O'Brien identifies a third tension between capitalism and caring: capitalist ownership undermines caring relations in the workplace. Capitalist managers generally place the goal of efficient production over work processes. Workers are forced to perform routinized and repetitive tasks without regard for their individual needs or social relations. Commenting on the development of Taylorism and other scientific management techniques in the United States, O'Brien writes:

Nothing could be further from the rationalization of the American workplace in the early twentieth than an ethic of care. Workers themselves were not viewed as individuals. Suggesting that employers should look into the faces of these individuals to discover their needs would have been considered outlandish. (2005: 84)

Although computers, robots, and other technological innovations now allow for a more individualized workplace, O'Brien notes that very little has changed in the organization of commodity production (88–91). Capitalist managers have simply used the new technologies to assert greater discipline over workers and to increase worker productivity (93–116).

Capitalism may finally be said to encourage an individualistic and selfish mindset that inhibits caring actions and attitudes among people. Bertell Ollman argues, for example, that people's experience of living, working, selling, consuming, and investing in market societies tends to generate 'a very distinctive view of the world' that is contrary to caring attitudes and practices:[11]

Human beings get thought of as atomistic, highly rational and egoistic creatures, whose most important activity in life is choosing (really, opting); because people choose without interference what they want (really, prefer), they are thought to be responsible for what they have (and don't have); the main relations between

---

[11] Ollman's critique is aimed not only at capitalist markets, but also at theories of market socialism. Insofar as socialism retains market processes, Ollman argues that it will still harbor the worst elements of capitalism.

people are taken to be competition and calculated utility, where each tries to use others as a means to his ends. . . . (Ollman 1998: 84)

In this capitalist worldview, people give very little consideration to the needs of others, let alone to helping them to meet their needs. Indeed, Ollman argues that in competitive market societies individuals tend to develop strategies for ignoring the needs of others since 'otherwise, learning that another person's need for food, a job, a home, or a sale in business is greater than one's own would inhibit one's ability to compete' (83–4). Market exchange further mystifies production processes so that consumers view products as already 'on the shelves' without considering the individuals who produced them and the conditions under which they were produced (86). Since individuals in capitalist societies relate to one another and the world around them primarily through commodities and money, they also tend to accord lower status to individuals who perform unpaid or poorly paid care work (100). In short, Ollman argues that the competitive market system encourages individuals to care very little about others and instead focus on their own consumption and happiness.

The four arguments listed above all point to the conclusion that some sort of socialist economy would be better at supporting caring activities than market capitalism. Socialism would seem better suited for steering economic production to meet human needs, supporting care work, promoting caring relations in the workplace, and fostering a caring mindset. This conclusion is, however, open to a number of criticisms. Each of the above arguments can be at least partially rebutted, and some of the criticisms leveled against capitalism can also be applied to socialism.

Regarding the first point, for example, although there is no necessary connection between capitalist production and the satisfaction of human needs, there is also no reason why capitalist production cannot be directed toward this end. If all people are guaranteed adequate resources for meeting their needs, then capitalist businesses will likely produce goods for them. While some goods may need to be publicly subsidized or directly manufactured by the government, most can be produced and supplied in highly efficient ways by market processes—just as long as all individuals possess adequate income to register their demand for them. In many cases, market demand may even provide a more sensitive mechanism for responding to individual needs than socialized production. As Polanyi argues, the market system itself is not to blame for the distribution of basic goods in capitalist societies. Rather, the blame lies with the misguided ideal of unregulated free markets. Private production and market exchange have been utilized in many societies throughout history without ignoring the needs of the poor. This problem arose only with the emergence of unregulated markets in the nineteenth century. While unregulated markets are certainly indifferent to human needs, a regulated capitalist market economy need not be. A capitalist market economy can be made to serve human needs by ensuring individuals the monetary purchasing power to express their needs and through other governmental regulations.

Held and Folbre themselves address the second criticism discussed above. While both writers argue that direct care services should be sheltered from market processes, neither suggests that the economy as a whole need necessarily be socialized. Held argues that direct care services should be socialized, but indicates that the rest of the economy might usefully continue to be governed by market competition (1993: 218–19, 224). Folbre claims that government regulation of caring activities may be sufficient in at least some cases to address the negative effects of a capitalist market system. Folbre further makes a point of noting that socialist economies are not necessarily better at supporting caring activities than capitalist ones (1996, 2001: 213–16). In line with traditional Marxist assumptions, Soviet planners, for example, devoted the lion's share of their society's resources to massive industrial and agricultural reforms while putting relatively little toward the support of caring practices. It is not obviously the case therefore that socialism automatically translates into more and better support for caring. Caring is an independent value that must be supported on caring grounds, whether under capitalism or socialism.

O'Brien's criticism is more difficult to rebut. In a competitive market economy, employers are likely to be more concerned with productivity and profits than with their workers' needs. Governments can intervene into labor processes (as most governments have done) to set minimal work standards for the decent treatment of workers. Yet, while these standards may prevent employers from exposing their workers to harmful work conditions or paying them unreasonably low wages, they generally do not ensure that employers will actually care for their workers in the ways O'Brien envisions. Some sort of worker control and ownership over production would seem necessary for achieving these aims (see also Schweickart 2002). It is not obvious, however, that promoting caring workplace relations should be a goal of care theory. Care theory, as I define it, aims only to ensure that all individuals can meet their biological and developmental needs and the needs of their dependents. As long as all individuals have real opportunities to work at adequately paying jobs, and policies exist (such as those discussed in Chapter 2) to support parenting, childcare, education, health care, and other caring activities, most individuals should be able to survive, develop, and achieve basic functioning even without a radical reform of the workplace. Reconstructing the workplace to promote worker control *might* help to make it a more caring place, but is not essential for ensuring that all individuals can survive and develop their basic capabilities.[12] From my perspective, then, O'Brien's call for a more caring workplace rests upon an overly broad definition of the nature and aims of caring. She understands caring to mean fostering good relations with others in all domains of society and responding to a broad array of their desires and interests. My own account focuses more minimally on helping individuals to survive, develop, and avoid pain and suffering so that they can function adequately in society. When caring is defined in this more minimal way, worker control and ownership does not appear to be a necessary element of a caring economy.

Finally, while an unregulated market economy would likely encourage individuals to develop an uncaring worldview, the same cannot be said of a regulated market economy, especially one that recognizes and supports caring practices. In countries where the government supports and accommodates caring practices, people generally express a strong sense of solidarity with others and a responsibility to help individuals with fewer resources (Rothstein and Uslaner 2005). Relations among people in capitalist societies are also not always as selfish and cold as Ollman portrays them. Even though market competition may encourage a certain amount of egoism and greed, everyday human relations under capitalism also involve a good deal of trust, honesty, consensus-building, and care (Nelson 2006). Alternatively, communism does not necessarily represent the panacea for human relations that Ollman portrays it as offering. Because communism replaces the market production and distribution of goods with social planning, it necessarily concentrates political and economic power in planning boards (however many and decentralized they may be) that determine what will be produced and how it will be distributed. Since the decisions of these boards would fundamentally impact the ability of individuals to survive and care for their dependents,

---

[12] Ollman argues that worker control in a market socialist society would actually achieve little in the way of improving worker relations and work processes, since competitive market pressures would drive workers to organize their workplaces to promote efficiency and productivity, much as current capitalist enterprises do (Ollman: 1998).

138

there would be great incentive for individuals to gain positions on them or curry favor with their members (Schweickart 1998: 13–14). Some measure of competitive relations would thus likely remain in communism, but only take a different form. Rather than competing for market share and profits, individuals would compete for political power and influence. In doing so, they would probably develop some of the same sorts of depersonalizing strategies for dealing with others that Ollman describes in market societies.[13]

In sum, then, market capitalism is not necessarily antithetical to caring, and socialism is not necessarily required for a caring society.[14] Rather, care theory remains relatively open toward different macroeconomic systems. There are some macroeconomic systems that are clearly unacceptable to care theory. An unregulated (or minimally regulated) free-market system, for example, would undermine direct care services and leave many individuals without the resources necessary to care adequately for themselves and others. A properly regulated market economy, however, need not have these consequences. Indeed, when one approaches economic questions from the perspective of care theory— asking whether individuals are able to meet their basic biological and developmental needs and provide adequate care to their dependents— abstract debates about the merits of capitalism, socialism, and communism become secondary. The important question is: Does the economic system adequately support and not unduly interfere with individuals' ability to give and receive adequate care? Since a number of economic systems may be capable of meeting people's needs and supporting caregiving, a variety of economic institutions are potentially compatible with care theory. Care theory ultimately favors whatever system may work best in a given context to ensure the adequate care and basic social functioning

---

[13] Marx, of course, predicted a great change in human nature following the communist revolution. It is hard to imagine a change so great, however, that individuals would become indifferent to decisions affecting their survival and basic functioning and the survival, development, and functioning of their children and loved ones.

[14] Other more indirect arguments might be made to support the case for market socialism from a caring perspective. Schweickart (2002) argues, e.g., that market socialism would better reduce unemployment and poverty and protect the environment than market capitalism can do. Since all of these aims are important from the perspective of care theory, his argument provides further support for the view that market socialism is most conducive to the aims and virtues of caring. Schweickart's arguments, however, rest upon the classical Marxist claim that capitalism requires artificially high levels of unemployment to maintain worker discipline, and that capitalism is necessarily expansionary. While unregulated capitalism may have these features, it is at least not obvious that a regulated market capitalism need function in this way. If Schweickart's arguments could be shown to be empirically true, however, they would lend support to the view that care theory is more compatible with a socialist economy.

139

of all individuals. More important from the perspective of care theory than the form of the economy are regulatory principles that guarantee the productive economy will support caring practices no matter what macroeconomic structure a society may adopt. As in the political arena, care theory thus shifts the debate about economic justice from a broad and oftentimes abstract concern with institutional form (capitalism vs. communism) to a focus on regulatory principles and policies. The principles and policies that form the core of care theory's account of economic justice are the subject of Section 3.4.

## 3.4. The Principles and Policies of a Caring Economy

A caring government will generally pursue four economic goals. First, it will promote a level of economic productivity and prosperity sufficient to meet the biological and developmental needs of its people. If the economy is not sufficiently productive, individuals will not be able to obtain the basic resources necessary to care for themselves and one another. A government might promote economic productivity in a number of ways, including enforcing contracts, discouraging corruption, supporting social infrastructures, and managing fiscal and monetary policy.

The government might achieve this first goal and yet many people could still go without adequate food, shelter, or education insofar as resources are poorly distributed. The second goal of a caring economic theory is therefore to ensure a minimally fair distribution of resources. The government should ensure that all capable individuals have real opportunities to work and obtain the resources needed to care for themselves and their dependents, and extend aid to individuals who are incapable of caring for themselves.

A third goal of a caring economic order is to promote individual responsibility. All capable individuals should be encouraged to work and/or care for themselves and others since society may not otherwise have sufficient resources to care for all of its members. Free riders not only drain resources away from those individuals who most need them but also fail to contribute to the web of social relations that sustain their lives.

The fourth goal of a caring economic theory is to support and accommodate direct care services and personal caring activities. The government should support and regulate direct care services such as education and health care, and should likewise provide support and workplace accommodations for personal caring activities, with the understanding that these services and activities have unique aims and virtues that are not adequately supported by either market or socialist goals. The aim should be to prevent economic processes and values from unduly interfering with the ability of individuals to give and receive adequate care.

Six economic policy principles follow from these goals. The six principles are interrelated and interdependent, and should not be considered in isolation from one another.[15] Together, they provide general guidelines for establishing and maintaining a caring economic order. The first principle is as follows:

(1) All individuals should have the opportunity to work at jobs that remunerate them at levels that are at least adequate to care for themselves and their dependents at a socially defined minimum threshold level.

This first principle incorporates elements from the first three goals discussed above. Governments should aim to promote a level of productivity sufficient to provide for all, they should support the broad distribution of resources, and they should encourage capable individuals who are not engaged in intensive personal care work to take part in commodity production. One way to achieve all of these goals is to ensure that adequately paying jobs are available to all individuals who are capable of performing them.

There are numerous ways for governments to promote jobs including: tax incentives for investment, consumer tax cuts, monetary policies that make credit cheaper and more accessible, fiscal policies that increase government expenditures, targeted wage subsidies designed to stimulate hiring, education and training programs, and a public jobs program (Gewirth 1996: 214–56; Rank 2004: 203–06). Governments might use some combination of any or all of these policies to ensure as much as possible that everyone has an opportunity to work. A government that simply heeded care theory's call for more public support for childcare, elder care, education, and other forms of care work would stimulate a great deal of job growth, since all of these fields are labor intensive.

A correlate to this first principle is workplace nondiscrimination and equal pay laws. If individuals cannot find work or are unfairly compensated because of discriminatory hiring and workplace practices, they will be impeded in their ability to obtain the resources necessary to care for

---

[15] Some of these principles would change somewhat under communism, since a fully communist economy would presumably exist without wages or taxes. The general commitments that stand behind these policies would nonetheless still apply.

themselves and their dependents, or may have to work longer hours and have less time to devote to care. Along these same lines, employers should also be required to make reasonable accommodations for workers with disabilities, since workplace accommodations may be necessary for providing these individuals with access to jobs and hence to the resources necessary to care for themselves and their dependents. While most accommodations are not costly, a government fund might be established to help employers to pay for any accommodations that are burdensome (O'Brien 2005: 140).

Individuals should also be guaranteed a decent minimum income for their work. Specifically, individuals who work full time (currently defined in most industrialized countries as working between 35 and 40 hours per week) should be able to obtain sufficient income to provide for themselves and their dependents at adequate levels. There are two main ways to ensure a decent income for all workers in a wage-based economy. One is by raising the minimum wage to ensure that individuals are paid an adequate amount. A second approach involves supplementing the incomes of low-income workers through measures such as the earned income tax credit (EITC). The EITC provides low-income workers with a partial subsidy (e.g. an additional dollar) for each dollar earned up to a certain point, and then is gradually phased out as the worker earns more money. The idea is to provide individuals with an incentive to work while ensuring that they are adequately compensated according to their needs and the needs of their dependents.[16] Governments might use some combination of minimum wage laws and EITCs (or other policies) to ensure that all working individuals are compensated for their labor at decent levels. For example, the minimum wage might be set at a level sufficient to ensure that individuals can earn enough money to care for themselves at a decent minimum, and then an EITC might be further provided to supplement the incomes of working individuals with children or other dependents.

The twin objectives outlined in this first principle—creating jobs and guaranteeing a decent minimum income—might seem to stand in tension with one another. Milton Friedman and others have argued that raising the minimum wage, in particular, provides a disincentive for employers to hire more workers and hence depresses job creation (Friedman 1982: 180–1). Empirical studies, however, have not borne out this claim: raises in the minimum wage have generally not negatively impacted

---

[16] For some examples of these plans, see Haslett (1994: 206–12) and Isbister (2001: 122–25).

employment (Card and Krueger 1995, 1999; Rank 2004: 197–200). In any case, governments might use the EITC to supplement incomes rather than raising the minimum wage if they so desire—a policy that Friedman himself originally proposed (Friedman 1982: 190–5). The question of how governments should attempt to ensure all capable individuals of access to adequately paying jobs is a policy matter that can ultimately be best decided in context and through experimentation. The goal, however, is clear: to ensure that everyone has an opportunity to work at jobs that reimburse them at levels sufficient to care adequately for themselves and their dependents.

Consistent with the goal of regulating the economy to support personal caring, care theory stipulates a second principle:

(2) Productive work should not unduly interfere with individuals' ability to care for themselves and their dependents.

This second principle is the flip side of the first one. Government should organize the economy not only so that it supports caring practices, but also so that it does not unreasonably interfere with them. There is something awry with an economic system that demands so much work from people that they have no time to care for themselves and their loved ones. When work unduly impedes caring, it undermines one of its core normative purposes.

The policy proposals that follow from this principle are pretty straightforward (Gornick and Meyers 2003). Governments should establish a maximum work day and work week so that individuals have sufficient time to rest and care for themselves and their dependents. They should likewise mandate publicly funded care leaves for new parents and individuals with sick or needy dependents so that they can take time off from work to care for these individuals. Individuals should also have access to long-term subsidized sick and disability leaves to care for themselves. A social fund similar to social security might be established to subsidize these leaves so that they are available to all and their costs are evenly distributed across society. Workers should also be guaranteed a number of days off from work each year for sick leaves or to care for their dependents. In short, personal care should be supported and protected from the demands of employers and the pressures of the workplace.

Another important measure for accommodating productive work to caring practices is flexible workplace scheduling (Bailyn 1993; Gornick and Meyers 2003; Williams 2000). Flexible scheduling includes a variety of options including: flextime policies that allow workers to begin or end their workdays earlier or later (e.g. 7 a.m. to 3 p.m. or 10 a.m. to 6 p.m); telecommuting where employees work at least part-time at home; job sharing where two individuals share the responsibilities, pay, and benefits of one job; and regularized part-time work that pays individuals and provides benefits at prorated amounts based upon a full-time employment scale (Williams 2000: 84–100). Flexible scheduling allows caregivers to arrange their work schedules so that they can spend more time with their dependents and be at home when, for example, children return from school. They also enable individuals who have primary responsibility for the care of dependent individuals to engage more easily in part-time productive work. Numerous studies have demonstrated that flexible scheduling can be beneficial not only for workers but also for businesses (Bailyn 1993; Williams 2000: 84–100). Where flexible scheduling has been introduced, it has tended to increase worker retention, loyalty, and productivity, and reduce absenteeism and employee costs. Joan Williams notes, 'Employers who dismiss scheduling flexibility as inefficient typically do not take into account how inflexibility costs them money. Surveys indicate that inflexible policies generate costs due to impaired job performance, absenteeism, and turnover, and that the costs of implementing a work/family program may be less than the costs of not having one' (2000: 88).

Despite the advantages of flexible scheduling, many companies may remain attached to traditional work schedules, and many employees may be hesitant to take advantage of flexible scheduling for fear of suffering the care penalty (Wiliams 2000: 94). Governments might encourage the implementation of flexible scheduling by temporarily offering tax incentives or taking other steps to encourage companies to offer their employees this option. Once flexible scheduling policies were more broadly instituted, other companies would be more likely to adopt them, and employees would likely feel more comfortable taking advantage of them.

The third principle of a caring economic theory addresses the conditions of work and specifically worker protections:

(3) No job or economic activity should unreasonably endanger or cause harm to workers or the environment.

Insofar as one of the primary reasons people engage in work is to obtain the resources necessary to care for themselves and their dependents, it makes no sense to permit work or production methods that unreasonably endanger workers or the environment. Dangerous and harmful work conditions may impair the ability of individuals to survive, sustain basic functioning, or care for others. Productive practices that pollute the air, waters, and land may likewise stunt the development of children or cause illness or death. Governments should therefore mandate workplace and environmental protection laws to support the care of all people. What exactly constitutes an unreasonable danger or harm is, of course, subject to debate and ultimately must be determined by researchers, policymakers, politicians, and citizens. In general, though, care theory supports a strict scrutiny test for any activities that threaten the immediate or long-term health, development, and functioning of human beings. Unless a dangerous occupational arrangement or harmful environmental practice can be shown to be absolutely necessary for satisfying basic human biological and developmental needs, it should be closely regulated or, barring some good justification, abolished. Economic activities that undermine or threaten human survival or decent caring contradict the fundamental normative purpose for which they exist.

While the first three principles of a caring economic theory all aim to subordinate productive work to the aims of caring, the fourth principle formalizes Held's and Folbre's concern that direct care services and personal caring activities be sheltered from the dynamics of market competition:

(4) Governments should ensure that direct care services and personal caring activities are adequately supported and fairly remunerated so that all individuals have access to affordable, quality care.

Many of the policies for supporting direct care services and personal caring practices were already discussed in Chapter 2 and above in discussing Held's and Folbre's theories. Individuals who care for others in need such as small children or disabled persons should be provided government subsidies to support their care work. The care sectors, including childcare, health care, elder care, disability care, and education, should be publicly regulated and subsidized to ensure affordable, quality care for all individuals. While it is probably not necessary, as Held suggests, for governments to socialize all the care sectors, they should establish regulations in market systems to prevent private providers from sacrificing quality care and take other steps to ensure that care workers are adequately trained and fairly compensated for their work. Suzanne Helburn and Barbara Bergmann suggest in this vein that governments should establish quality control measures for all childcare centers, and set a special minimum wage for childcare work somewhat higher than the national minimum wage in order to offset the care penalty and reduce turnover among workers (2002: 202). Childcare centers would have to meet these quality and wage requirements in order to be eligible for public vouchers or subsidies. Similar measures might be enacted to address the low quality of services, poor pay, and high turnover rates in other care professions. Decent pay is essential in these fields not only for attracting and retaining competent care workers, but also for paying individuals fairly according to their qualifications and the importance of their work. Market competition can be useful in promoting efficiency and innovation, but should not be allowed to undermine good care.

In addition to subsidizing direct care services and personal caring activities, care theory also directs governments to provide temporary unemployment or emergency assistance to otherwise capable individuals who may not be able to care for themselves and their dependents. This is the fifth principle of a caring economic theory:

(5) Capable individuals who cannot support themselves and their dependents should be provided temporary assistance until they can achieve adequate levels of self-support. Individuals who are incapable of working should likewise be supported.

This fifth principle institutionalizes the social practice that Polanyi claims was central to nearly all premodern economic systems: to provide decent care to all individuals unless the group itself is faced with shortages (Polanyi 2001: 48, 171–2). While premodern societies may have supported this goal out of sense of communal solidarity, care theory suggests that individuals in modern societies should do the same out of their sense of obligation to care for others.

Even in a prosperous economy, many individuals are likely to experience temporary periods of unemployment or under-employment where they may have difficulty meeting their needs and caring for their dependents. David Rank estimates, for example, that by age 75, over 58 percent of individuals in the United States will have lived in poverty for at least one year (Rank 2004: 62–4). Governments should extend subsidies to these individuals to help them through these periods of hardship. The goal should still be to encourage full employment for all capable individuals not engaged in intensive personal care work. As such, governments might sponsor a public jobs program for those who cannot find work, offer job training classes, or sponsor other employment programs. Yet some individuals simply may not be able to find adequate work for some periods and may require some temporary assistance.

Workfare programs, which require aid recipients to perform at least some work in exchange for benefits, are also a legitimate means within care theory for moving capable but unemployed individuals into remunerative work—given certain conditions. These programs should provide individuals with at least an adequate level of remuneration (as discussed above), make exceptions or provisions for individuals with dependents (such as providing them with subsidized parental leaves and childcare subsidies), provide them with an opportunity to develop their work skills through training programs or education, and avoid making unreasonable demands regarding the type of work to be done and the length of the commute to their workplaces. If individuals must commute two hours each way to their place of employment, for example, their opportunity to care for themselves and their dependents will be markedly diminished.

The final principle of a caring economic theory addresses the need for raising public revenues to support caring activities. Since in communist societies all resources are publicly owned and distributed, this principle would apply only to market- and wage-based economies. In market- and wage-based economies, moral guidelines for raising revenues, or tax rates, can be best determined through a just entitlement theory. A just entitlement theory identifies levels of personal property that individuals might rightfully claim for themselves and their dependents before contributing to the general care of others. For the just entitlement principle outlined below to yield fully caring results, a society would have to be able to generate sufficient resources to meet at least an adequate threshold of care for all its members.[17] To the extent that a society cannot generate sufficient resources, it will be less than fully caring regardless of whether it is market-based or communistic. In less than ideal circumstances, it might be suggested that a communistic distribution of resources would be preferable to an individual entitlement principle, since the whole group would (at least hypothetically) absorb shortages under communism rather than placing the burden on particular individuals. The argument for communism under less than ideal circumstances rests, however, on the judgment that it is better to allow all the people to starve halfway than to permit half the people to starve. The alternative view is that it is better to allow half the people to meet their basic needs adequately

---

[17] Rawls argues in this vein that moderate scarcity represents a basic precondition for justice (Rawls 1999: 109–12). If natural and other resources are not available to support at least the survival and basic functioning of individuals, then he argues that schemes of cooperation must inevitably break down.

than to condemn everyone to a life of stifling poverty. Both situations are equally tragic, and it is not obvious that either one is clearly more caring than the other. Where trade-offs are less stark—requiring that ninety-nine people sacrifice one-hundredth of their barely sufficient resources in order to allow one person to survive—then the sacrifice would seem warranted. But one need not turn to communism to support this measure. Care theory's just entitlement principle should be understood to contain a special exemption in dire circumstances that justifies miniscule decreases below the adequate threshold of caring in order to support a basic threshold of caring for some individuals who would otherwise not survive. In general, under conditions of moderate scarcity, care theory's principle of just entitlement may be stated as follows:

(6) Individuals are entitled to retain that portion of their resources necessary to care adequately for themselves and their dependents. They are further entitled to retain some amount of resources above this basic subsistence level in order to support their pursuit of some conception of the good life. Individuals might also be allowed to retain additional resources insofar as it serves as an incentive to generate more social resources for individuals in need. Individuals are finally entitled to keep all resources not necessary for the care of others.

In the remainder of this section, I discuss and defend this principle, and then conclude by comparing this account of just entitlement with Robert Nozick's libertarian entitlement theory.

Individuals are most basically entitled to keep whatever resources they lawfully earn, own, or acquire up to the point necessary to provide themselves and their dependents with adequate care.[18] The justification for this principle follows from the distribution of our caring duties outlined in Chapter 1. Although we all have general duties to care for others in need, we are primarily responsible for the care of ourselves and our immediate dependents because we can usually care most attentively, responsibly, and respectfully for them. Except in dire circumstances, redistributing resources away from individuals who lack sufficient resources to care for themselves and their immediate dependents is likely to result in inefficiency and a lower level of care for all. All individuals should therefore be exempted from taxation until their resources clear a minimum threshold

---

[18] For the sake of simplicity, I focus here on general taxation guidelines without delving into questions of how exactly the government should tax personal income, wealth, inheritance, business activity, and the like.

necessary for providing themselves and their dependents with adequate food, water, clothing, shelter, medical care, childcare, dependent care, and education. Insofar as some of these goods are publicly provided (e.g. health care and education), the personal income needed to meet this threshold level might be set at lower levels.

Individuals are further entitled under care theory to retain some resources above this subsistence level in order to pursue their ideal of the good life, including the development of their own or their children's complex capabilities.[19] Once again, this principle of just entitlement follows from the argument in Chapters 1 and 2. Care theory, as I have argued, is an incomplete moral and political theory. It specifies a decent moral minimum for our relations with others but recognizes the existence of other goods in life that individuals may consider equally important to caring, including play, knowledge, religion, artistic expression, and pleasure. Since caring for others cannot be shown in all cases to be clearly more important than these other goods, individuals are entitled under care theory to devote some portion of their resources to these other goods even at the cost of caring for others. This is not to say that a fully caring society would be one where some people spend resources on religious pursuits or pleasure while others starve, but rather that a fully caring society requires a level of productivity that can provide for the basic needs of all individuals while also giving individuals some opportunity to pursue their conception of a good life.

Peter Singer argues against this view that expending resources on any higher goods when some individuals cannot even meet their basic needs is immoral (Singer 1993: 264–88). Singer's argument rests, however, on the assumption that his account of preference utilitarianism should predominate over all other moral views. Care theory cannot justify the absolute predominance of caring values over all other moral views and thus adopts a more modest approach. (Singer, of course, likewise cannot justify the moral predominance of utilitarianism over all other values; he merely asserts his view as comprehensive.) Because we all have caring obligations to others regardless of our conception of the good life, care theory suggests that individuals who devote some resources to the pursuit of the good life

---

[19] Care theory does not necessarily presume a liberal society where individuals are free to pursue diverse conceptions of the good life. It is possible to envision a more communitarian caring society in which individuals pursue the good life collectively, say, by practicing a common religion. In such a society, a similar distributional principle would nonetheless apply. The government might legitimately expend some money on the collective ideal of the good life, e.g. building Synagogues, Churches, or Mosques, even if it were not capable of helping all people to meet their basic needs.

should also devote some portion of their excess resources to the care of others in need. A caring government is thus justified in taxing at a partial rate the income or wealth of individuals above what they need to care adequately for themselves and their dependents.

Some additional excesses of income and resources might be further allowed insofar as they provide individuals with an incentive to be more productive and contribute more to the pool of resources available for caring. Rawls's difference principle endorses this sort of arrangement (Rawls 1999b: 53). Rawls argues that social and economic inequalities ought to be permitted insofar as they redound to the benefit of the least advantaged member of society. Care theory's difference principle is somewhat more broad and general than Rawls's, suggesting that differential incomes should be allowed insofar as they serve to encourage people to generate more resources for supporting the care of individuals in need. In any case, care theory generally follows Rawls in allowing for differential incomes as a means for promoting greater productivity. It should be noted, however, that there appear to be some limits to income incentives of this sort. Several studies have found that, at least among high-income individuals, high tax rates have no significant effect on work effort or productivity (Easterly 2001: 234–5; Goodin 1988: 231–2). Individuals in high income professions tend to remain productive even when taxed at high rates for the sake of status, power, prestige, and other nonmonetary rewards. At lower income levels, however, overly arduous tax rates might have a depressing effect on productivity and reduce the resources available for caring. Some income inequality thus might be allowed in a caring society in order to foster more economic productivity and innovation and hence a greater supply of resources and quality services to support caring practices.

Individuals are finally entitled under care theory to keep that portion of their surplus income or resources not necessary to support the care of others. Care theory is not an egalitarian theory in the sense that it aims to limit income differentials as an end in itself. It justifies taxing the income and resources of individuals only for the sake of supporting the care of others. Once the government has accumulated sufficient resources to support caring practices at adequate levels, individuals should be allowed to keep whatever additional resources they earn or possess. Since the costs of caring are fairly high, income and wealth differentials are nonetheless likely to remain within a moderate range in a caring society.

In general, then, care theory supports a tax scheme that exempts individuals from taxation up to the point necessary to provide adequate care for themselves and their dependents, and then taxes some portion of their income or wealth beyond this point. In practical terms, a progressive tax scheme with a fairly high basic exemption would probably best fulfill these requirements. Such a tax scheme would leave untouched the resources that individuals need to care for themselves and their dependents, allow lower income individuals a greater percentage of their small excess income or wealth to devote to their pursuit of the good life, and leave higher income individuals with a smaller percentage but larger real monetary amount to devote to their life goals, thus providing some incentive for higher productivity and innovation. Within this tax scheme, individuals might be given partial tax credits for their charitable contributions to private care organizations or even for their charitable care work insofar as a trustworthy scheme of accountability could be established. Care theory does not require that all social caring take place through governmental channels. There would, nevertheless, have to be a limit on these tax credits, since government action would still be necessary to coordinate the distribution of resources for caring, to provide support for individuals in need, and to provide some basic goods such as protection, clean water, and a safe environment.

Care theory's entitlement principle is very nearly the mirror-opposite of Robert Nozick's libertarian theory. Nozick's entitlement theory states that individuals are entitled to keep all the resources that they have justly acquired through contracts, gifts, and other uncoerced exchanges (1974: 150–3). If people are willing to pay Wilt Chamberlain an exorbitant sum to watch him play basketball, Nozick argues, there is no injustice in allowing Chamberlain to keep all his excess wealth. On the contrary, it would be unjust to tax Chamberlain's justly earned income. Why, Nozick asks, should Chamberlain be required to give up some of his hard-earned income to subsidize the lives of others? (160–4).

Care theory answers: Because if it were not for the care of his parents, teachers, coaches, and others, Chamberlain would never have become a great basketball player. And if not for the care of other parents, teachers, coaches, aunts, uncles, and others, there would be no fans to appreciate his talents. Care theory would remind the hypothetical Chamberlain that his basketball talents would mean nothing outside society, and that society would not exist without the web of caring. Since we all depend on this web of caring for our survival and social existence, we are all morally obligated to contribute to its maintenance and reproduction insofar as we are able to do so. We are all entitled to retain the resources necessary to care for ourselves and our dependents at adequate levels and some additional resources to pursue our conception of the good life. But to claim for ourselves all the resources we have been able to acquire in and through society is to forget the debt we owe to society and the caregivers who sustain and reproduce it. Nozick apparently forgets that no man or woman is an island. We are all deeply dependent upon others and society for our survival, development, and well-being, as well as for our opportunities for gain within the productive economy. If we have surplus income, we owe at least some of it to help support the parents, teachers, childcare workers, and others who sustain human life and make economic activity possible.

A caring theory of economic justice is ultimately very different from liberalism, libertarianism, socialism, or communism. Care theory does not aim to promote individual autonomy, social equality, worker control, or unexploited labor, but instead to assure all individuals access to the resources and support necessary to care adequately for themselves and their dependents. To this end, it supports adequately paying jobs for all; workplace accommodations for caring; workplace and environmental protections; subsidies for direct care services and personal caring; temporary support for individuals in need; and a tax scheme that encourages both personal responsibility and caring for others. Altogether, the principles and policies of a caring economic theory aim to direct and regulate economic activities so that they support and do not impede caring practices.

## 3.5. The Challenge of Globalization

Even if one finds attractive the goals and principles of a caring economic theory, they might no longer seem feasible in a globalized economy. Companies can now move their manufacturing and telecommunications operations from countries with high minimum-wage laws and strict workplace and environmental regulations to countries with lesser or no minimum-wage laws and safety and environmental regulations. This global 'race to the bottom' makes it extremely difficult for governments to maintain the sorts of policies and regulations necessary to maintain a caring economic order. It therefore might seem that a caring economy is no longer a real possibility.

In considering the viability of a caring economic system within a global economy, it is first important to make a distinction between the empirical processes of globalization and the ideology of neoliberalism (Steger 2002).

Globalization refers to the increased integration and interdependency of economies and societies around the world. While the scope of globalization has sometimes been exaggerated, it does appear to be a real and significant phenomenon (Hirst and Thompson 1999). In recent years, world trade has grown dramatically, international financial transactions have increased, and transnational corporations have moved many of their manufacturing and telecommunications operations from industrialized to developing countries (Steger 2002: 21–8). We may not now (or ever) live in a fully globalized world, but the world economy is becoming more integrated. Neoliberalism, by contrast, refers to a set of economic and political doctrines promoting the ascendancy of largely unregulated or free markets. Neoliberals have seized upon the real processes of globalization to argue that markets have triumphed over governments, that there is little governments can do to control markets, that governments must accede to market pressures by cutting services and encouraging free trade, and that free markets will in any case benefit everyone (Steger 2002: 43–80). While these claims have been put forth with great persuasiveness in popular works (see, e.g., Friedman 2000), there is little empirical evidence to support them, and a fair amount to refute them. Governments and international organizations still have a good deal of power over market processes. Indeed, to the extent that markets are now ascendant over governments, it is largely because governments and international organizations such as the International Monetary Fund, World Trade Organization, and World Bank have vigorously pressed for free-market policies over the past three decades (Falk 1999; Weiss 1998). It is widely recognized now, too, that the blanket imposition of neoliberal policies on developing countries has not benefited all people but instead provoked financial crises, exacerbated income inequalities, and brought on a good deal of hardship (Hahnel 1999; Stiglitz 2002). Just as in the nineteenth century, to quote Polanyi, 'the gearing of markets into a self-regulating system of tremendous power was not the result of any inherent tendency of markets toward excrescence, but rather the effect of highly artificial stimulants administered to the body social', so today the ascendancy of markets is not inevitable or natural but the result of policies enacted by governments and international organizations (Polanyi 2001: 60). And just as the attempt to establish self-regulating markets in the nineteenth century threatened to annihilate 'the human and natural substance of society' and provoked dangerous countermovements, so the same is happening today (Polanyi 2001: 3). Yet globalization does not necessarily mean neoliberal globalism. The world economy can still be made to serve social goals, and particularly, the goals of human caring.

There exist numerous proposals for regulating the world economy according to social goals, and it is not my intention here to outline a comprehensive approach to global market regulation (Beneria 2003: 161–9; Falk 1999; Greider 1997: 316–30; Hahnel 1999: 82–108; Held 1995: 221–86; Steger 2002: 135–50; Stiglitz 2002: 214–52). Instead, I wish only to highlight a few policies that might help to promote a more caring world economic system. One important step toward this goal would be the ratification of regional and global treaties on minimum wages, worker protections, and environmental standards. Wage scales could be calibrated to the different living standards of different countries, and worker protection and environmental policies might be varied somewhat depending on circumstances, but the idea would be to guarantee all workers at least subsistence wages, safe working conditions, and a clean environment. The governments of developing countries have sometimes objected to these sorts of proposals on the grounds that they might deter companies from moving into their countries. Yet productive work that pays less than subsistence wages, endangers workers, or unduly degrades the environment hardly seems to be in any people's interests. Since developing countries generally have lower costs of living than developed countries, they would still enjoy a comparative advantage under this plan in the form of lower—albeit now decent—wages. Meanwhile, by setting a floor on global wages, workplace conditions, and environmental standards, the governments of industrialized countries could elevate the 'race to the bottom' and slow the movement of manufacturing work to developing countries, thus giving their citizens more time to develop new productive industries.

Since regional and global treaties on wages, worker protections, and environmental standards would likely slow the economic development of third world countries, they would necessarily have to be complemented by development aid to these countries—at least, that is, if the people of industrialized countries wish to behave caringly toward the people in these countries. In Chapter 4, I more fully discuss our caring duties to others in international relations. Here, though, a few points can be made. A caring development program aims most basically to help people in other countries to satisfy their needs for food, sanitary water, adequate housing, basic medical care, education, and other basic needs. While helping people to meet their basic needs may not be sufficient for stimulating economic development, these goals do seem a necessary prerequisite to any more comprehensive development program (Streeten 1981). Where people are undernourished, sick, or have little real opportunity to develop their basic capabilities, economic productivity will be low regardless of capital investment, debt relief, or any other measures aimed at stimulating economic development. People must be able to stand before they can walk, and currently, too many people in poor countries can barely bring themselves to their feet each day. Helping people to meet their vital biological and developmental needs, too, represents an important stimulus to economic development. As Amartya Sen argues, investments in labor intensive care services such as health care and basic education not only provide many people with training and jobs, but also facilitate the development of the human capabilities that are essential for long-term economic growth (Sen 1999: 35–53).

A caring economic program also offers industrialized countries a good strategy for coping with the dislocations caused by a globalized economy. Public investments in caring services such as health care and education generally mean a more capable and productive workforce. More capable and productive individuals, in turn, are more likely to attract jobs, innovate, and contribute new goods and services to the global economy (Reich 1992). Investment in care work also represents a means for broadly distributing income throughout society and stimulating domestic demand. Since care work is labor-intensive, public investment in the caring professions means more jobs for more people. If more people have jobs and more income to spend—and spend it mostly on basic needs and developmental goods—they will stimulate demand for more basic goods (Greider 1997: 320–8). Since the global market is not now, and probably never will be, a seamless web, increased domestic demand is likely to translate into more domestic production and business enterprises. People still have to acquire goods at local stores and businesses, after all, and caring services cannot very easily be outsourced to other countries. Investment in care work can thus stimulate domestic economic productivity and job growth. At the very least, it seems more likely to do so than offering tax breaks to the rich, since wealthy individuals may invest in any number of (not necessarily socially beneficial) enterprises anywhere in the world.

These comments about care and globalization are admittedly sketchy. A full discussion of globalization and the steps that might be taken to control it lies beyond the scope of this book. Here I wish only to emphasize three points relevant to my argument. First, the global ascendancy of markets is not inevitable. It is possible through national policies and international treaties to subordinate global markets at least in part to the aims of caring. Second, a caring domestic economic policy is viable. The increased globalization of the world does not necessarily mean that governments must cut spending on domestic programs and loosen workplace and environmental regulations. In order to maintain caring policies, however, they do need to cooperate with other governments to establish international labor, wage, and environmental standards. Third, a caring economic theory may actually offer a more effective strategy for addressing the challenges of globalization on a national and international level than neoliberal policies. Investments in care work not only promise a better quality of life for people, but also provide the basic conditions for long-term economic growth and prosperity.

## 3.6. Conclusion

Care theory provides a rather commonsensical framework for thinking about economic justice. Most people work primarily for the sake of caring for themselves and their dependents, and caring practices sustain economic production and reproduce society. Even more basically, we should all be able to recognize a moral duty to support economic institutions and policies that provide all individuals with real opportunities to work and care for themselves and others. Most societies throughout history have at least implicitly recognized the interdependency of care work and commodity production, and subordinated commodity production in part to the aims of caring. Many contemporary societies, however, seem largely to have forgotten this lesson. Care theory aims to redress this imbalance by partially re-subordinating economic activity to the aims and virtues of caring.

Virginia Held and Nancy Folbre have outlined proposals for support- ing direct care services. This chapter has extended their arguments to show more broadly how productive economic activities might be orga- nized to support and accommodate everyday caring practices throughout society. A caring theory of economic justice aims to ensure that every- one has access to the economic means necessary to care for themselves and their dependents; that economic activities do not unduly interfere with the ability of individuals to care for themselves and their depen- dents; and that direct care services and personal caring activities are adequately supported. As noted above, care theory does not require eco- nomic institutions and policies to be organized exclusively around caring aims and virtues. People might also wish to pursue other goals through their economic institutions. Support and accommodation for caring practices would nonetheless seem a basic goal of any just economic order. If an economic order does not support human caring, it is hard to understand why human beings should support it. It is also an open question whether human beings can continue to survive and function over the long run without giving more attention to the caring practices that sustain us.

# 4

# Care Theory and International Relations

People sometimes draw a fairly sharp distinction between the moral rules that apply to domestic politics and those that apply to international relations. While it is generally accepted that rules of justice should govern our relations with fellow citizens, or compatriots, our moral duties to people in other countries are often considered quite minimal. The realist school of international relations most fully embraces this perspective, arguing that governments should set aside moral considerations in international relations and conduct their foreign policies primarily in terms of self-interest and power. By contrast, cosmopolitan political theorists argue that our duties of justice extend at least in part beyond our home societies to encompass individuals in other countries (Beitz 1979; Brown 2002; Jones 1999; Pogge 2002; Singer 2002). Care theory enters the debate between realists and cosmopolitans on the side of the cosmopolitans. Because our obligations to care for others are rooted in the universal claims we make on others for care, our duty to care for others is necessarily universal in scope. Even though we are justified in showing some preference in caring for our compatriots (see Chapter 1), we nonetheless also have duties that extend to the care of distant others. The purpose of this chapter is to describe what exactly these caring duties entail in the domain of international relations.

Two important books have already taken up the issue of caring for others in international relations: Sara Ruddick's *Maternal Thinking* (1989) and Fiona Robinson's *Globalizing Care* (1999).[1] Ruddick's book is grounded in the practice of mothering and the aims associated with it: preserving life, fostering growth, and training for social acceptance. While acknowledging that actual mothers often support wars and militarism, Ruddick

---

[1] For more limited discussions of care theory and international relations, see also Gould (2004) and Held (2006: 154–68).

argues that the *logic* of maternal thinking favors a nonviolent peace politics (Clement 1996: 92). The goal of a nonviolent peace politics is 'to create conditions of "peace" in which people can self-respectfully pursue their individual and collective projects free of the structural violences of poverty, tyranny, and bigotry' (Ruddick 1989: 161). The central strategies for achieving this goal are the renunciation of violence and weapons, resistance to unjust and harmful policies, a willingness to forgive and reconcile with enemies, and a desire to avoid battle (160–76). For Ruddick, these strategies form the core of a caring international agenda, though she also applies them to domestic and inter-personal relations. Despite her advocacy of a nonviolent peace politics, Ruddick importantly distinguishes her position from pacifism (137–9). She argues that one should be suspicious of violence even in the best of causes because of its high physical, moral, political, economic, and other costs. 'But—and here is the primary difference with pacifists—a sturdy suspicion of violence does not betoken absolute renunciation... Although she will never celebrate violence, a peacemaker may herself act violently in careful, conscientious knowledge of the hurt she inflicts and the costs to her as well as her victim' (138). For Ruddick, violence is always a tragic last resort; it is always harmful and costly and should be avoided as much as possible. Nonviolent peacemakers will therefore strive to avoid the need for violence by establishing a just peace and devising strategies of nonviolent reconciliation and resistance whenever possible (172).

In *Globalizing Care* (1999), Robinson echoes and extends many of Ruddick's themes. She argues that caring for others means not only meeting their needs but also working to identify and change social institutions that make individuals needy and dependent in the first place (1999: 110). She calls this approach a 'critical ethics of care:'

What this means is not simply that the powerful must learn to "care about" the suffering and the destitute in what could possibly—although not necessarily—become a paternalistic act which preserves existing power relations. It means that those who are powerful have a responsibility to approach moral problems by looking carefully at where, why, and how the structures of existing social and personal relations have led to exclusion and marginalization, as well as at how attachments may have degenerated or broken down so as to cause suffering (46).

Building upon this approach, Robinson argues that a caring approach to world poverty would 'require that the powerful—states, NGOs (non-governmental organizations)—adopt strategies which pay attention to the relationships and attachments, both within existing communities and between members of organizations in the North and peoples in the South, and explore how those relations might perpetuate, or lead to solutions concerning, levels of poverty and well-being' (153). More generally, she suggests that international aid groups should move beyond the 'model of partnership', where powerful groups distribute goods to needy individuals without redistributing decision-making power, in order to embrace a 'model of partnering' based 'on respect for control by the local partner' and 'close face-to-face interaction between organizations and their constituencies so that ideas and policies are shaped in the crucible of everyday practice rather than in the upper echelons of remote and rule-bound bureaucracies' (Robinson 1999: 159–60). The goal is to empower individuals to care for themselves and their dependents and to forge more egalitarian cross-cultural relationships.

Ruddick and Robinson identify some important goals for care theory in international relations. Both agree that governments and international organizations should shift the focus of international relations from the 'moment of decision-making' to the structural conditions of peace and well-being, and each further suggests strategies for fostering more caring relations among peoples (Robinson 1999: 144). For Ruddick, this involves a commitment to nonviolent peacemaking, and for Robinson it means critically assessing our relationships with others and developing more egalitarian partnering relationships. The arguments of both writers, however, remain at a fairly general level. Neither says very much about how exactly peoples and states ought to go about establishing the background conditions of peace, or proposes anything like a body of rights for institutionalizing caring relations among people worldwide. Much of what it means to care for others in international relations therefore remains ambiguous.

Robinson, in particular, resists formulating her theory in terms of rights and obligations, asserting that normative international relations theories already focus too much on justice principles (1999: 3). The problem with these theories is that they tend to promote 'a depersonalized, distancing attitude toward others' that distorts 'the real contexts of relationships among particular persons' (Robinson 1999: 8, 37–42). By her estimation, care theory is better framed as a 'moral phenomenology' emphasizing the dispositions or virtues necessary to respond to individuals and situations in attentive and responsive ways' (7, 37–42). While Robinson's dispositional approach may be useful in describing how to care for others in international relations, it does not tell us enough about whom or what we should care about. Should we form partnering relationships with all groups or only some, for example, and should we support all the projects that local groups might propose or prioritize some over others? Framed so abstractly, Robinson's theory provides little practical guidance for policymakers, activists, and the general public in thinking about what it might mean to care for others abroad.

In this chapter, I develop a more concrete account of a caring international relations theory that identifies the rights and polices that follow from human beings' duty to care for others. The first half of this chapter develops a human rights framework based upon care theory. This framework avoids some of the central shortcomings of other international rights frameworks, and more generally provides a standard of justice that should be reasonably acceptable to people from diverse cultural and religious backgrounds. The second half of the chapter outlines some specific strategies and policies for enforcing human rights abroad. In outlining these strategies, I pay special attention to the moral hazards that accompany efforts to care for distant others. In Section 4.4, I further outline a form of just war theory based upon care ethics and discuss the conditions under which care theory justifies military interventions into other countries for humanitarian purposes.

The central purpose of this chapter is to develop a caring international relations theory that can stand alongside liberal, natural law, utilitarian, and other normative approaches to international relations as a distinctive perspective on international justice (Mapel and Nardin 1998; Nardin and Mapel 1992). A second important purpose is to highlight the valuable contribution that care theory can make to debates about international justice. In response to recent cultural challenges to human rights, theorists have sought to develop international justice frameworks that should be reasonably acceptable to people from diverse cultural, religious, and moral backgrounds (Gewirth 1996; Habermas 1984, 1987, 1998; Rawls 1999). Care theory offers an account of human rights and international justice that plausibly meets these requirements. By rooting human rights and international justice in human beings' universal dependency upon one another for care, care theory outlines a normative international relations theory that applies to all human beings regardless of their culture, religion, or morality, and can provide substantive guidance for cross-cultural dialogue among diverse peoples about the moral treatment of all human beings. A final purpose of this chapter is to outline a number of concrete policies and strategies for translating the commitments of care theory into actual practice. Theories of international justice are all well and good, but may have little effect on the actual practice of international relations unless they also specify the practical policies that follow from them.

## 4.1. Care Theory and Human Rights

While human rights stand at the center of most discussions of inter-national justice, their moral status remains a contentious issue. Jack Donnelly, to cite only one example, argues that all foundational justifi-cations for human rights are ultimately question-begging (See also Rorty 1989). ' "Foundational" arguments operate within (social, political, moral, religious) communities that are defined in part by their acceptance of, or at least openness to, particular foundational arguments' (Donnelly 2003: 18). According to Donnelly, attempts to ground human rights in divine law, human nature, the inherent dignity of the human person, or other sources will be more or less persuasive to individuals only to the extent that individuals already accept these foundations as normative. By Don-nelly's account, there is no foundation for human rights except for human beings' 'decision to act as though such "things" existed' (2003: 21). *constructivism?*

Donnelly argues that the lack of foundations for human rights is not a problem in the contemporary world because human rights have become 'a hegemonic political discourse' (2003: 38). The governments of nearly all states have agreed to respect and enforce the Universal Declaration of Human Rights (UDHR) and other international human rights treaties. Moreover, human rights are today 'a standard subject of bilateral and mul-tilateral diplomacy', and 'most national societies are also increasingly pen-etrated by human rights norms and values' (2003: 38). Donnelly further suggests that 'there is an international overlapping consensus on the Uni-versal Declaration model,' by which he means that most people can find moral justification for most rights contained within the UDHR in their own comprehensive moral, cultural, and religious beliefs (2003: 40–41).[2]

Donnelly is surely correct to emphasize the prevalence of human rights discourse in the world today but overstates the substantive agreement that exists about these rights (Freeman 1994). As he himself admits, the practical consensus on human rights is 'often very shallow—*merely* verbal' (1989: 42) Many governments have agreed to follow the UDHR only at their discretion, and some have ratified international human rights

 *response*

---

[2] The idea of an overlapping consensus is borrowed from Rawls (1996, 1999). Significantly, though, Rawls argues that an overlapping consensus supports a much narrower set of rights in international affairs than those contained in the UDHR.

treaties with explicit reservations. Donnelly, too, understates the force of cultural challenges to the UDHR (Donnelly 2003: 107–23).

The leaders of China, Singapore, and several other Asian and African states have argued that a number of the political and civil rights contained in the UDHR are incompatible with the collectivist values of the majority of people in their societies (Bell 2000; Donnelly 2003: 71–123; Hamdi 1996; Kausikan 1993; Tang 1995; Vincent 1986: 37–57; Zakaria 1994). Some Islamic leaders and scholars likewise maintain that human rights guaranteeing equal treatment to women and religious minorities conflict with Islamic law (An-Na'im 1990; El-Affendi 2001; Hamdi 1996; Mayer 1991; Rishmawi 1996; Tibi 1994). Government leaders have no doubt sometimes used cultural arguments in cynical ways to justify their power and interests, but many cultural challenges are not so easily dismissed (Bell 2000; Pollis 1996; Pollis and Schwab 1979; Renteln 1990; Rorty 1989). Adamantia Pollis writes:

The passage of time has not diminished the salience of the early claim that in many societies—Asia, Africa, Eastern Europe (including Russia), and the Middle East—the liberal doctrine of human rights does not speak to the people's world view. The ontological foundations of their cultures and society, often reinforced by the political regime on matters such as the nature of man/woman, her/his identity, and the person's relatedness to others and to society, differ in significant ways. (Pollis 1996: 316)

Chris Brown notes in a similar vein that, whether or not the UDHR is ultimately biased toward Western liberal values, its articles do at least require a Western-style liberal democracy: 'all political systems that are not liberal-democratic are delegitimized by the international human rights regime' (Brown 2002: 190).

The broad array of rights enumerated in the UDHR and international rights treaties also create problems for generating an overlapping consensus on them. The UDHR enumerates rights to life, liberty, and security; freedom of thought, expression, assembly, and religion; political participation; property; work, rest, and leisure; an adequate standard of living; education; nationality; and participation in the cultural life of one's community. The International Covenants on Economic, Social, and Cultural Rights and Political and Civil Rights (1966) further extend these rights to encompass self-determination, protection of minority cultures, and several other entitlements (Donnelly 2003: 24). The breadth and diversity of these rights means at the very least that international human rights advocacy will be diluted, and some basic rights may be ignored in the quest to assure freedoms or self-determination for individuals (Agarwal 2005). Potential conflicts between a number of these rights— for example, between rights to self-determination and security, property and redistribution, cultural expression and individual freedom—further erode their legitimacy (Ignatieff 2001: 20, 22–30). If not all human rights can be equally enforced and respected, then governments will necessarily have to choose to enforce some rights over others, and no government or people can unhypocritically criticize others for failing to respect all human rights.

Given the (at least) nominal support that the UDHR already enjoys among governments and the pivotal role it plays in international discussions on human rights, it would be foolish to suggest that this document should be discarded altogether. However, if human rights are to be more broadly respected and enforced across the world, it would seem important to be able to identify a generally acceptable moral foundation for them as well as a cogent set of basic rights within the UDHR that deserve priority over other rights. Care theory can plausibly offer a solution to both of these challenges.

Caring practices include everything we do directly to satisfy human beings' vital biological needs for food, water, shelter, clothes, rest, a clean environment, basic medical care, and protection from harm; to foster and maintain the basic human capabilities for sensation, mobility, emotion, imagination, reason, communication, affiliation, literacy, and numeracy; and to help individuals to avoid or alleviate unwanted or unnecessary pain and suffering. The ultimate goal of caring is to help individuals to survive, develop, and achieve social functioning as much as possible without pain and suffering. Care theory's approach to human rights closely resembles the basic needs approach outlined by theorists such as Paul Streeten (1981) and Henry Shue (1996) (see also Stewart 2006). Streeten and Shue argue in a manner similar to care theory that international justice should focus on helping individuals to satisfy their basic needs for food, sanitary water, shelter, protection, health care, and the like. Care theory nonetheless supplements the basic needs approach in a couple of ways.

Most basically, care theory provides a richer and deeper philosophical foundation for the basic needs approach. As Amartya Sen has argued, the basic needs approach is not 'deeply founded' (1987: 25). Streeten rests his basic needs theory on the intuitive idea that helping individuals in need is a fundamental moral duty. Shue argues in a somewhat more sophisticated manner that 'if there are any rights (basic or not basic) at all, there are basic rights to physical security' and subsistence, since physical security and subsistence are necessary for the enjoyment of all other rights (1996: 21). Shue's defense of rights nonetheless remains hypothetical: he does not attempt to show that human beings actually have a right to any protections or goods, but argues only that if human beings have any rights, they should have rights to satisfy their basic needs. Care theory supplements the basic needs approach by attaching a theory of obligation to it.

The full argument for our obligation to care for others was outlined in Chapter 1, but can be briefly recapped here. We all make (or at least have made or will make) claims on others to help us survive, develop, and function. No one could survive, develop, or function during infancy and childhood, grave illness, disability, frail old age, or other periods of particular hardship without the care of other human beings. We all further depend upon the care of others to sustain the social network that we require to survive and function. In attempting to justify our claims for care on others, we have all implicitly appealed to the general moral principle that capable individuals should care for individuals in need when they are able to do so. Because we have all necessarily appealed to this moral principle, we may all be said to recognize it as valid; and if we all recognize this principle as valid, then we all should—out of a sense of consistency and morality—recognize and respond to the claims of other individuals in need for care when we can help them. We behave hypocritically and inconsistently when we refuse to care for individuals whom we are capable of helping, and violate our own implicit moral beliefs.

Care theory's account of moral obligation can thus provide a more satisfactory philosophical justification for the basic needs approach. We should help other individuals to satisfy their basic needs not simply for intuitive reasons or out of some vague regard for human dignity but because we have all claimed care from others in meeting our own needs, and more generally committed ourselves to the general moral principle that caring for others in need is morally right. Because the moral principle of caring for others does not make any distinction between compatriots and noncompatriots, we should care for all other human beings in need when we are capable of doing so wherever they may live.

Care theory further supplements the basic needs approach by addressing a number of criticisms that, fairly or not, have been leveled against it (Reader 2006). Sen, for example, has criticized the basic needs approach for focusing too much on goods and services and not enough on 'what people can *do* or can *be*' (Sen 1984: 510). Without some notion of valuable human ends, the meeting of needs can become an end itself regardless of its effect on human capabilities (Sen 1987: 24–6). The narrow focus on goods and services also fails to appreciate that the 'same capabilities' can be supported 'by more than one particular bundle of goods and services', and alternatively, that one particular bundle of goods and services may not be sufficient for helping all individuals to achieve the same capabilities (1984: 513–14). By Sen's account, the basic needs approach also runs the risk of treating individuals paternalistically. In the basic needs approach, human needs are sometimes treated as self-evident commodities rather than as something that individuals in need should be able to define and specify for themselves (1984: 514).

Whether or not these criticisms are valid when directed against the basic needs approach, they do not apply to care theory.[3] Care theory embeds the goal of meeting needs within the larger goal of helping individuals to meet the valuable human ends of survival, development, and social functioning. It likewise remains open to the possibility that different bundles or combinations of goods and services may be able to achieve similar results in different societies and for different individuals. What matters from the perspective of care theory is that all individuals are able to meet their needs at levels adequate to support their survival, development, and functioning. Because caring for others necessarily involves the virtues of attentiveness, responsiveness, and respect, care theory further avoids concerns about paternalism (White 2000). If individuals, groups, or governments are to care effectively for others, they must engage with them to discover what they need, how they can be helped, and how their existing capabilities can be utilized to help them meet their needs.

While care theory incorporates elements of the capabilities approach, it also departs from existing interpretations of this approach in a couple of ways. Sen orients his capabilities approach around the goal of enhancing individual freedom (1999). Martha Nussbaum grounds her theory 'in the Marxian/Aristotelian idea of truly human functioning' and 'an intuitive idea of a life that is worthy of the dignity of the human being' (2000: 5, 13). Nussbaum, as distinct from Sen, further specifies a list of capabilities for truly human functioning that include: living out a human life of normal length (clause 1); enjoying bodily health and integrity (clauses 2 and 3); developing and freely using one's senses, imagination, emotions, and reason, and experiencing and producing self-expressive works and events of one's own choosing (clauses 4 and 5); exercising practical reason

[3] Reader argues that these criticisms are not, in fact, decisive or in some cases even accurate, and further addresses Sen's other criticisms of the basic needs approach (Reader 2006).

and forming a personal conception of the good life (clause 6); engaging in various forms of social interaction (clause 7); living with concern for animals, plants, and nature (clause 8); being able to laugh, play, and enjoy recreational activities (clause 9); and exercising control over one's political and economic life (clause 10) (Nussbaum 2000: 78–80).

While Sen's and Nussbaum's capabilities theories have gained a great deal of attention in recent years, the grounds upon which they base their theories are highly contentious. Few societies outside the West place the premium on individual freedom that Sen does, and despite Nussbaum's claim that her theory is 'free from any specific metaphysical grounding', it is difficult to see how one can arrive at her account of 'truly human functioning' without some metaphysical premises about human nature and the good life—especially given her reluctance to associate her theory too closely with empirical or anthropological data (5). Care theory largely avoids these problems by grounding the duty to care for others in the empirically verifiable dependency of all individuals on the care of others. We have duties to care for others because we all necessarily depend upon others for care. Care theory also avoids controversial claims about what constitutes a truly human life by focusing more narrowly on what Nussbaum calls the 'basic capabilities' or 'innate equipment of individuals that is the necessary basis for developing the more advanced capabilities, and a ground of moral concern' (84). Since it can be plausibly assumed that all individuals wish to survive, develop their innate capabilities, and achieve and maintain basic social functioning, care theory's framework more plausibly provides a universal standard of justice than Nussbaum's extensive list of capabilities (Okin 2003).

Care theory can ultimately be translated into a theory of international human rights. Because all individuals in need can justify their claims on others for caring by appealing to the general moral principle that capable individuals should care for individuals in need, they can validate their claims for care against one another. Individuals' claims for care are therefore justifiable or valid rights claims (Feinberg 1970). Care theorists have generally been wary of adopting the language of rights on the grounds that traditional liberal rights can be distancing and depersonalizing (Gilligan 1982; Noddings 1984; Robinson 1999). Yet there are many ways to understand rights, and there is no reason why a conception of rights cannot be developed based upon our caring obligations to one another. The body of rights outlined below, for example, lists the obligations that human beings owe to one another based upon our universal dependency in meeting our biological and developmental needs.

Most of the rights listed below have been discussed in the la⌐
ters. They are formulated more abstractly here, however, to a⌐
the possibility of multiple realizability in different cultures a⌐
(Nussbaum 2000: 77). While the general aims of caring rem⌐
across cultures, the specific means of caring for others may be quite
different in different cultures, especially when considering the best means
of providing support for childcare, elder care, health care, and so forth.
The list also contains some rights not explicitly discussed in the last two
chapters, but relevant to caring in the world at large. More rights might be
added to the list insofar as they can be shown to be necessary for caring,
but a basic list of caring rights includes the following:

(1) All individuals have the right to physical security, including protections against bodily assault, sexual assault, child physical and
sexual abuse, domestic violence, unwarranted police or military
violence, torture, cruel and unusual punishment, and arbitrary
arrest and detention. Consistent with these protections, all individuals should also enjoy rights to due process and a fair trial.

(2) All individuals have the right to food, sanitary water, clothing,
shelter, basic medical care, a clean environment, and rest at levels
adequate to survive, develop, and function. Governments should
provide all individuals with real opportunities to obtain these
goods, and provide support to individuals who cannot reasonably
obtain these goods by their own efforts. *physical needs*

(3) All individuals have the right to the personal and social care
necessary to develop and sustain their basic capabilities for sensation, mobility, emotion, imagination, reason, communication,
affiliation, literacy, and numeracy at levels adequate to function in
society. The right to personal and social care should be understood
to include access to adequate care during childhood, sickness,
disability, and old age, and a basic education.

(4) All individuals have the right to work and earn a living sufficient to
satisfy the biological and developmental needs of themselves and
their dependents.

(5) All individuals have the right to care for their dependents
and themselves without undue interference from work or other
sources. Maximum daily and weekly work limits should be
established so that individuals are able to rest and care for themselves and others. Women should be provided maternity leaves and

guaranteed the opportunity to return to their jobs at the same pay at the end of their leaves. Individuals should be offered subsidized work leaves to care for new children, sick relations, or themselves. Some number of sick or personal leave days should be guaranteed to all workers each year for the care of self or others.

(6) All individuals have the right to a safe workplace, including occupational safety requirements and environmental protections. Regulations should be placed on child labor, in particular, to ensure that children have an opportunity to develop their basic capabilities.

(7) All individuals have the right to unemployment and disability insurance to help them meet their basic needs and care for others during periods of temporary hardship.

(8) All individuals have the right to protection against discrimination on the basis of race, sex, sexual orientation, religion, caste, ethnicity, or national origin in matters directly affecting their ability to give or receive care, including their ability to work, obtain resources or services, or form relationships.

(9) All individuals have the right to a responsive government, including institutional channels for expressing their needs to government officials and opportunities to exercise some control over local policies affecting their lives.

(10) All individuals have the right to enter into relationships free from coercion. Slavery and indentured servitude as well as forced and underage marriages should be prohibited.

Most of these rights follow fairly self-evidently from the aims and virtues of caring. Caring means most basically protecting individuals from physical harm and unwarranted detention so that they can survive, develop, and function in society without unwanted suffering or pain. Caring further means helping individuals to satisfy their basic biological and developmental needs and providing support for them during periods of special dependency. Governments should therefore provide all individuals with environmental protections and basic infrastructure goods such as sanitary water and sewage systems that are necessary for their survival and health. Governments should likewise provide support for direct care services such as education, health care, childcare, and elder care (adapted, of course, to the diverse circumstances of different peoples), and further offer subsidies and support for individuals who cannot meet their basic needs. Work opportunities and wage laws are important so that individuals can obtain the resources necessary to care for themselves and others, and work regulations are necessary to ensure that productive processes do not unduly interfere with the ability of individuals to give and receive adequate care. Anti-discrimination laws are also important in this regard, since discriminatory practices may make it difficult for individuals to obtain the resources necessary to care for themselves and others or otherwise threaten their survival or basic functioning. Individuals should further be able to express their needs and concerns to the government and have some control over the design and implementation of local programs so that public programs address their particular needs. Individuals should finally be protected against coercive relationships that may threaten their lives, the development of their basic capabilities, or their ability to care for themselves. In sum, care theory guarantees all individuals access to all the protections, goods, and services necessary to support their survival, development, and basic functioning.

Primary responsibility for securing the rights of people falls upon the governments of countries, since they are usually best positioned to organize collective policies to meet the particular needs of their people. If governments cannot secure their people's rights, however, the international community assumes this responsibility. We all have residual responsibilities to care for distant others when their governments cannot or will not do so. This notion of residual responsibilities represents an important departure from the UDHR, which calls upon states to enforce the rights of their own citizens but says nothing about inter-state responsibilities (Donnelly 2003: 34). Under care theory, individuals and governments have a responsibility to provide resources and other forms of support to distant people when distant peoples and their governments are unable to support their survival, development, and functioning by their own means.

While the idea of a universal obligation to care for others might seem an overly demanding ethic, there are reasonable limits to it. Individuals and governments are responsible for caring for distant others only after they have provided adequate care for their families and the people in their home countries. This partiality is justified on the grounds that individuals can usually use their resources most effectively to care for individuals who are close to them and share social institutions with them. It makes little moral sense to direct resources away from individuals in our immediate environment who need our care in order to care less effectively for distant others. Individuals and governments are further justified in retaining some portion of their excess resources to use in pursuing their conception

*[handwritten marginal note: Justifications for international intervention]*

of the good life. If all resources were put first and foremost to caring, then caring would consume almost all resources, and individuals would have little opportunity to pursue other conceptions of the good life. Caring for others, however, cannot be justified over and above all other ideas of the good life as the single most important aim of human life. Care theory therefore recognizes the justifiability of devoting some resources to the pursuit of other goals even at the cost of caring for others. In many cases, caring for others in distant countries may further involve not so much a donation of resources to distant others as a willingness to change national and international laws and policies that hinder the ability of people in poor countries from satisfying their needs (see below).

The duty to care for distant others therefore does not require individuals and governments to sacrifice their own care or all other goods for the care of distant others. It does, however, place a duty on all people to provide resources and otherwise take actions to help distant others when they are able to do so. What this means in practice will, of course, vary according to the circumstances of different societies, but as a minimal baseline, it would seem that most individuals in most industrialized societies should be able to devote at least one to two percent of their above poverty income each year to caring for distant others in need, and governments in wealthy countries might devote at least one to two percent of their gross national product to humanitarian foreign aid. Even this small donation of aid would represent a great increase over the amount most individuals and governments currently give, and would go a long way toward saving the lives and fostering the healthy development of millions of people who currently die each year from malnutrition and disease.[4]

Although there is a good deal of overlap between the framework of caring rights and the UDHR, care theory departs from the UDHR in important ways. Many of the classical liberal rights contained within the UDHR, for example, are only weakly represented or not included in the list of caring rights.[5] While care theory endorses the right of

[4] There might be some concern that caring for distant others could exacerbate population growth and contribute to environmental and other problems. In general, though, when people are provided good care and opportunities to care for themselves, population levels begin to level off or even decline (see Sen 1999: 189–226; Singer 1993: 235–41).
[5] Care theory departs from recent liberal approaches to international justice on similar grounds (see, e.g., Buchanan 2003a; Rawls 1999; Tan 2000). Most liberal authors premise their theories—whether explicitly or implicitly—on contentious ideals such as equal respect or autonomy. Care theory grounds international norms in the caring practices that are universally necessary for human survival and reproduction. Many liberal theories of international justice, too, emphasize in one way or another principles such as self-determination, national

people to a responsive government, it does not require a democratic or representative government based upon 'periodic and genuine elections which shall be by universal and equal suffrage' (UDHR, article 21). There are numerous ways to organize a responsive government other than a representative or democratic government based upon universal and equal suffrage. A meritocratic bureaucracy with a strong ethic of public service might be just as responsive, or even more so, than a representative democracy; a parliament of appointed leaders from diverse groups throughout society might also be highly effective at addressing people's needs (Bell 2000: 53–4, 164–8, 279–336). Periodic elections and universal suffrage may be useful in some contexts for securing responsive government, but they are not necessary for this purpose. Care theory favors any number of arrangements as long as they assure that government officials remain attentive and responsive to their people's needs.[6]

Care theory also lends only weak support to religious and civil freedoms. Rather than a right to freedom of religion (UDHR, article 18), care theory supports only a right to protection against religious discrimination. Individuals ought to be protected against harassment, arrest, imprisonment, workplace discrimination, and the like based upon their religious beliefs. It would be oppressive and uncaring for a government to prevent individuals from meeting their needs or those of their dependents because of their religious beliefs. It would likewise be uncaring for a government to prevent individuals from practicing religious beliefs that they consider essential to a meaningful life. However, if a government or people chooses to provide public support for one particular religion or places some prohibitions on the practice of religion—such as rules against proselytizing—this is not necessarily contrary to the principles of care theory. The care of all individuals can be secured without necessarily guaranteeing all individuals a broad right to religious freedom. Care theory similarly offers only weak support for the rights to freedom of speech and assembly (UDHR, articles 19 and 20). If governments are to remain responsive to people's needs, they must allow individuals some freedom

autonomy, democracy, or civil freedoms, but not necessarily the positive duties of peoples to help others meet their basic needs. Care theory, by contrast, focuses on our duties to help others meet their biological and developmental needs, but for the most part sets aside questions about self-determination and freedom as matters to be decided by different peoples according to their different conceptions of the good.

[6] As noted in Chapter 2, while Amartya Sen has shown that democracies are generally effective at avoiding famines, they are not necessarily better at responding to the everyday needs of their people (Sen 1999: 154, 160–1; see also Bell 2000: 36).

of expression. At the very least, individuals must be able to express their needs and concerns to the government. However, individuals need not necessarily be allowed a right to protest, speak badly about governmental officials, or publish divisive news stories. Free expression is justified within care theory only insofar as it is necessary to support a responsive and caring government.

In addition to the liberal rights discussed above, care theory does not support rights to nationality, cultural expression, and self-determination. In most cases, these rights are not necessary to survival and basic functioning.[7] There may, of course, be situations where individuals can only assure their survival and functioning by asserting their autonomy from an existing government. In these cases, care theory does support something like a right to nationality or self-determination. However, it does so in these cases not because it supports a right to nationality or self-determination per se but rather because nationality and self-determination may be necessary in some cases to enable groups of individuals to care adequately for themselves and their loved ones.

In sum, care theory may be said to offer a distinctive approach to human rights. Rather than resting human rights on appeals to human dignity (the UDHR)—or freedom (Sen), the idea of truly human functioning (Nussbaum), individual autonomy (Buchanan), or equal recognition and respect (Rawls)—care theory rests human rights on the universal dependency of all human beings on the care of others and the moral obligations that follow from it. In turn, care theory supports a more cogent set of human rights than those contained in the UDHR. While the caring framework of rights is no doubt still quite extensive, it at least organizes all human rights around the one fundamental moral aim of supporting human survival, development, and social functioning. Finally, care theory is also more open to reasonable differences among people about the proper aims and nature of government than the UDHR and many other human rights frameworks. The caring body of rights does not prescribe the form or final ends of governments, but rather identifies a basic set of rights that all people should be able to recognize as fundamental to the decent moral treatment of others regardless of the particular form of their governments.

*[handwritten margin note: dependency focused rather than individualistic]*

---

[7] As Buchanan argues, in many cases, the rights of individuals to survival and basic development can be best secured by working for accommodation within existing states (Buchanan 2003a). Ignatieff similarly notes that movements for self-determination can sometimes be detrimental to basic survival and developmental rights of people (Ignatieff 2001: 22–30).

## 4.2. Care Theory and Cultural Diversity in International Relations

Care theory ultimately provides a standard of justice that should be reasonably acceptable to people from diverse cultural and religious backgrounds. In fact, many of the world's people already appear to support something akin to the caring rights listed above. International surveys and conferences, for example, demonstrate broad support for caring rights among the world's people. Drawing upon the Beijing Fourth World Conference's *Platform for Action* and World Bank's *Voices of the Poor*, Susan Okin notes that most individuals agree about certain basic human rights such as the right to physical security; 'having the ability to feed, clothe, and shelter themselves and their children, as well as to provide them with health care and education necessary for their avoiding poverty in the future'; having access to safe drinking water and other basic infrastructure goods; having access to land, credit, and jobs sufficient to meet their basic needs; and having influence over the events around them (Okin 2003: 301–2, 306–10). Most succinctly, 'They want to be able to live free from hunger, thirst, exposure to the weather, ill health, humiliation, and fear' (310). In other words, individuals from diverse cultures and backgrounds agree about the fundamental importance of rights to care for themselves and their dependents. By contrast, Okin finds far less agreement and unmitigated support for rights to free expression, free religious practice, democratic governance, and other liberal goods.

Nearly all the world's major religions similarly support the moral duty to care for others in need (Lauren 1998: 5–9). Judaism contains numerous injunctions to care for others such as Isaiah's call for followers 'to share your bread with the hungry, and to bring the homeless poor into your house' (58:7). The Christian Bible is similarly rife with exhortations to feed the hungry, heal the sick, clothe the naked, and care for the vulnerable and needy. One of the central pillars of Islam is charity toward those who are less fortunate than oneself. Buddhism emphasizes the virtues of charity and compassion toward others. Confucianism stresses familial duties and an impartial concern for the suffering of others, and imposes a responsibility on rulers to provide for their people's well-being (Bell 2000: 50, 77, 96). Similar principles can be found in most of the world's other major religious traditions. Most people can therefore find support for the body of caring rights within their own religious and cultural traditions.

The same cannot so clearly be said, once again, about liberal rights to free expression and democracy.[8]

Even most critics of human rights agree in principle that human beings should enjoy rights to life and basic social functioning (Bell 2000: 28–9). Most challenges to human rights focus more narrowly on the legitimacy of rights to democratic participation, equality, freedom of speech, freedom of assembly, freedom of religion, and other typically Western liberal rights. Care theory avoids most of these disputes by supporting only the rights that most everyone already recognizes in principle. It does not press for individual equality or freedom, make strong claims for civil and political rights or religious freedoms, or assert that democracy is the only legitimate form of government. It promotes only those rights necessary for individual survival, development, and basic social functioning. In this regard, it meets many human rights critics on their own grounds. In 'Asia's Different Standard' (1993), Bilahari Kausikan argues that many people in East and Southeast Asia are not so much interested in Western human rights or democracy as 'effective, efficient, and honest administrations able to provide security and basic needs with good opportunities for an improved standard of living' (37). Lee Kuan Yew, one of the most outspoken proponents of the Asian values thesis, similarly endorses a list of governmental principles very close to the body of caring rights listed above. He defines the principles of good government in the following terms:

a.  People are well cared for, their food, housing, employment, health.

b.  There is order and justice under the rule of law, and not the capricious, arbitrariness of individual rulers. There is no discrimination between peoples, regardless of race, language, religion. No great extremes of wealth.

c.  As much personal freedom as possible but without infringing on the freedom of others.

d.  Growth in the economy and progress in society.

e.  Good and ever improving education.

f.  High moral standards of rulers and of the people.

g.  Good physical infrastructure, facilities for recreation, music, culture and the arts; spiritual and religious freedoms, and a full intellectual life. (Quoted in Bell 2000: 186)

[8] On this idea of constructing a defense of human rights out of existing religious and moral doctrines, see Cohen (2004). I suggest that it is much easier to find support for care in existing religious and moral doctrines than it is to find support for democracy, freedom of speech, and other liberal rights.

Care theory certainly does not endorse all the policies Lee Kwan Yew enacted as Prime Minister of Singapore, but his support for this list of governmental principles does indicate his willingness to endorse the body of caring rights. More generally, care theory's approach to rights is more compatible with the communal orientation of many Asian and African peoples than the UDHR and liberal rights frameworks. By emphasizing the interdependency of individuals in meeting their needs, care theory situates rights in the web of social relations and supports family and communal forms of care much as many Asian and African peoples do (Brown 2002: 196).

Care theory might seem to avoid one sort of human rights bias only by propagating another. Care theory's list of rights might be readily accepted by Lee Kuan Yew and many of the world's peoples, but might seem grossly inadequate from a liberal perspective. For many liberals, democratic participation, religious toleration, and free expression are the very essence of human rights. Yet care theory offers only weak support for these liberal rights. While it is certainly understandable that liberals might object to care theory on these grounds, the charge of bias here rests on a misunderstanding of the nature of care theory's rights. Care theory supports the rights it does because they are essential to support adequate caring. Adequate caring, in turn, is necessary to support human survival, development, functioning, and the pursuit of any conception of the good life. Even liberals are thus implicitly committed to the rights of care theory (though many liberal theorists have ignored them) since caring precedes and is necessary for freedom, equality, and democracy. In this regard, it is misguided to say that care theory is biased against liberalism. It merely supports a more basic set of rights than liberalism does— specifically, rights to caring activities and goods that make liberalism (and all other political arrangements) possible. Liberals might advocate a broader list of human rights than care theory does by arguing that the best society should encompass not only caring rights but also democracy, free speech, self-determination, and the like. Almost invariably, however, their arguments will make appeal to some contentious claims about the good life that not everyone may be willing to accept. Care theory leaves aside claims about the best life for human beings and instead focuses on the human rights that underlie all conceptions of the good life, and that all people should be reasonably willing to endorse.

Even though most people may express principled support for care theory's framework of rights, some governments or peoples may nonetheless engage in practices that violate these rights, and justify their practices through appeal to cultural or religious traditions. Women, for example, might be exposed to honor killings or deprived of educational opportunities on the grounds that these practices are necessary to ensure the integrity of the culture or are condoned by religious law. Individuals who argue on behalf of such practices, however, support a self-refuting thesis. All human beings share common biological and developmental needs that must be met through the care of others. This is true of women no less than men, of racial minorities no less than racial majorities. Each of us has called upon other human beings to help us meet our needs, and in the process, tacitly endorsed the idea that capable human beings ought to help other human beings to meet their needs. Individuals who support practices that cause harm to others or deprive them of the opportunity to develop their basic capabilities thus violate their own implicit moral beliefs. They refuse to extend to others the very care that they demand for themselves as dependent beings.

Some governments or people may nevertheless argue that their religious or cultural practices should take precedence over the goal of guaranteeing adequate care to all individuals. Yet, as discussed in Chapter 2, the rights of caring morally trump the claims of religion and culture. Before there can be any religion or culture, there must be caring practices that make human life and society possible. Religious or cultural practices that violate the rights of caring thus contradict the moral preconditions of their own existence. They place the reproduction of a certain way of life above the practices necessary for the reproduction of human life itself. Care theory also places the rights of individuals above group values and goals. Since we claim care from others as individuals, it is to individuals that we owe care. This interdependency of individuals is what ultimately binds groups together and reproduces them over time. Since all groups depend upon individual care for their very existence, the care of individuals rightly has precedence over any collective values or goals that may interfere with it.

While some peoples or governments may simply ignore the rights of certain individuals to adequate care, most are likely to profess a sincere commitment to caring for others, but disagree about its meaning. Western peoples may consider harsh initiation rites such as female genital operations and ritual scarring as abusive, while the people who perform these rites may consider them supportive of their children's development and social functioning. Alternatively, non-Western peoples may regard the child rearing practices of Western peoples as abusive and uncaring. Traditional Turkish women were alarmed, for example, when a Western anthropologist allowed her daughter to play in a small pool of water

*[margin note: isn't this contradictory to the basis being human dependency?]*

*[margin note: disagreements between cultural ideas of care]*

on warm days. Believing that children are easily chilled and should not be bathed too frequently, they regarded the anthropologist's action as jeopardizing the health, and perhaps survival, of her child (Korbin 1982: 259–60; Olson 1981: 113–14).

Although care theory allows for some reasonable differences among people about the best way to care for others, it also offers a practical standard for determining the minimally adequate care of individuals. Since the aim of caring across cultures is to help individuals to survive, develop, and enjoy basic functioning, the morality of different practices can be judged according to whether they actually help individuals to achieve these ends, or at least do not impede their ability to do so. The Turkish women's concerns about the Western anthropologist's child rearing practices can be shown through observation and empirical study to be unfounded, since bathing or swimming outside on warm days is usually not harmful to children. Alternatively, Western (and many non-Western) people's concerns about female genital operations appear to be well-founded. A Kenyan study reported that more than eighty percent of girls who undergo female genital operations report at least one medical complication from these procedures, and other reports estimate that significant numbers of girls die from them (Williams 2000: 264). More generally, these operations deprive women of their sensory capabilities. Care theory draws the line at any practice that clearly involves threats to the survival, bodily integrity, development, and health of children and other dependent individuals. Female genital operations on young girls are wrong from the perspective of care theory because they deprive girls of sensation and feeling, cause them suffering, and threaten their survival and long-term health.

The acceptability of a number of other cultural practices, including ritual tattooing and scarring, harsh initiation rites, polygamy, and other practices are more open to debate. These practices do not necessarily threaten the lives, development, or functioning of individuals, but they may do so. Care theory addresses these issues by offering a cross-cultural standard for evaluating them. The question that care theory asks us to consider is: Does the practice hinder the ability of individuals to satisfy their basic biological needs, impede their ability to develop and maintain their basic capabilities, expose them to unnecessary and unwarranted suffering and pain, or most generally hinder or blight their lives and functioning? If the answer to this question is yes, then the practice should be disallowed for moral reasons. If the answer is no, then care theory is morally neutral toward it.

Different societies may ultimately establish somewhat different stand-ards of adequate caring based upon their peoples' different understand-ings of harm and the requirements of social functioning. While ritual scar-ring may seem abusive in one society and hinder a person's opportunities to work and care, it may represent a welcome rite of passage in another society and provide a person with power and prestige. Whether or not a particular practice is caring will usually depend to some extent upon the requirements of social functioning in a particular society. Nonetheless, as noted above, there are certain moral absolutes in care theory. Practices that threaten the lives or blight the development or functioning of indi-viduals are never justifiable under this theory.

Where different groups or individuals disagree about the morality of a practice, care theory endorses cross-cultural dialogue oriented around the aims of caring (Parekh 2000). Critics might challenge some law or practice on the grounds that it undermines the ability of individuals to satisfy their biological or developmental needs. Defenders might respond by arguing that the law or practice does not actually impede individuals' survival or development in their social context. In all cases, the discussion returns to the question of whether a particular practice threatens the survival, development, or functioning of individuals or causes them unwanted or unnecessary pain. Suppose, for example, we regard some groups' marriage laws or policies toward women as harmful. We might initiate a dialogue with them in the following way:

We think that all individuals should enjoy rights to life, development, basic functioning, and freedom from suffering. Yet, your law X appears to have the effect of depriving women and girls of some of these rights. We care about them and are therefore concerned about X.

Our discussants might respond: We, too, agree that life and functioning are good things and try to guarantee as much as possible that all individuals in our society have rights to life, development, basic functioning, and freedom from suffering. But you misunderstand the nature of law X and how it functions in our society. X actually helps to secure the survival and basic functioning of girls and women by protecting them against abuse, sexual assault, and other dangers.

We might reply: Yes, but at what cost? The girls and women in your society are made vulnerable to other forms of abuse and manipulation, and many cannot even obtain the basic resources they need to survive by their own efforts. Might not women be protected against abuse, sexual assault, and other dangers without subjecting them to the oppressive regulations of X?

The conversation may go back and forth from this point. While some debates may not achieve any clear resolution, care theory at least provides an internal foothold within different cultures for challenging and discussing the justifiability of various practices. Since everyone should be able to acknowledge the morality of caring, all sides should at least be able to agree in principle about the nature of human rights and goals of justice. Individuals who refuse even to acknowledge the morality of caring not only set themselves against the practices necessary to sustain human life and society, but in many cases also violate some of the most basic dictates of their religious or cultural beliefs.

## 4.3. Strategies for Caring

It is one thing to identify the general aims of care theory in international relations, but quite another actually to care for distant others. Because we may have limited knowledge about the needs of distant others, limited understanding of how our actions might affect them, and limited control over their political institutions and policies, it is easy for even the most well-intentioned efforts to care for distant others to go awry. Over the last decade, scholars and activists have highlighted some of the dangers associated with long-distance caring, or what is more commonly known as humanitarian assistance (Barrett and Maxwell 2005; de Waal 1997; Gourevitch 1998: 256–74; Kennedy 2004; Maren 1997; Wenar 2003). While acknowledging that many humanitarian aid initiatives have successfully averted impending crises, these critics argue that many efforts have also been ineffective or even harmful to people. Large influxes of cheap or free food aid into countries over extended periods of time can drive down prices for locally grown crops, undermine domestic farming, and breed dependency on foreign food aid (Barrett and Maxwell 2005). Government officials and local leaders may appropriate foreign food or monetary aid to distribute as patronage to their supporters, and some aid programs have fueled crime, sexual exploitation, and violence. Thomas Weiss lists only some of the recent failings of humanitarian aid in the following inventory:

The 'dark side' of humanitarian action would include: food and other aid usurped by belligerents to sustain a war economy (e.g. in Liberia); assistance that has given legitimacy to illegitimate political authorities, particularly those with a guns economy (e.g. in Somalia); aid distribution patterns that have influenced the movement of refugees (e.g. in eastern Zaire); resource allocations that have promoted the proliferation of aid agencies and created a wasteful aid market that encourages parties to play organizations against one another (e.g. in Afghanistan); elites that have benefited from the relief economy (e.g. in Bosnia); and resources that have affected strategic equilibriums (e.g. in Sierra Leone). (1998)

These empirical considerations raise further questions about what it means to care for distant others. In the abstract, we might acknowledge our moral duty to help distant others to meet their basic needs, develop and sustain their basic capabilities, and alleviate their suffering. In practice, though, we cannot always fulfill this duty simply by sending food or blankets overseas or providing monetary aid. In some cases, simple-minded approaches to caring may actually do more harm than good. Among care theorists, Nel Noddings has been most sensitive to these issues. Because of the difficulties and hazards involved in caring for distant others, she has even appeared to suggest at times that there is very little we can do to help individuals abroad (Noddings 1984: 86, 1992: 110–16). While this view seems overly pessimistic, her point is nonetheless well-taken. Caring for others means not just intending to do good but actually achieving good outcomes.[9] No matter how good our intentions may be, our actions can hardly be considered caring if they fail to help people to meet their needs or, even worse, exacerbate their misery. If we cannot act in ways that will actually help others to meet their needs, we might be best advised to do nothing at all.

In light of these concerns, two general principles can be suggested as guidelines for determining when and how we should attempt to care for distant others. Both principles follow from the nature of caring itself:

(1) The goal of caring should be to enable individuals and families as much as possible to care for themselves or to return as quickly as possible to a condition where they can care for themselves without outside support. No policy or program should function to promote the long-term dependency of individuals on foreign aid or undermine the stability and safety of a region.

(2) Local peoples and governments should be involved as much as possible in the formulation and implementation of programs intended to help them. Donor governments and aid organizations should form partnering relationships with local peoples and governments that allow the latter wide scope in determining the programs and policies best suited to meet their needs (Robinson 1999).

[9] Michael Slote, by contrast, argues that intentions should carry more weight than consequences in assessing the morality of actions within care theory (Slote 2001).

The first of these principles derives from the aims of caring. Although caring aims most directly at meeting the basic biological and developmental needs of people, its ultimate goal is to help individuals to graduate (whenever possible) to a state of mature social functioning where they can care for themselves and others.[10] Activities that leave potentially capable individuals in a state of perpetual dependency are not so much caring as a form of malignant paternalism that makes the perpetuation of caring itself the goal of the activity. The second principle is rooted in the virtues of caring. One must be attentive, responsive, and respectful toward others in order to care effectively for them. At a broad social level, these virtues translate into the requirement that donor governments and groups ask potential aid recipients to identify and prioritize their needs, respond to their suggestions, and acknowledge and utilize their capabilities. Most generally, they should engage in the sort of partnering relationships described by Robinson. Partnering relationships are not only necessary to care effectively for distant others, but also help to mitigate concerns about paternalism in long-distance caring (Narayan 1995).

These two principles have important implications for providing long-distance care. We might generally think about caring for distant others in three different ways: (*a*) direct foreign aid and human rights advocacy, (*b*) capacity building, and (*c*) changes in international law. In pursuing these strategies, the overriding goal (following from the two principles listed above) should be to shift the actual delivery of care to local levels and enable individuals as much as possible to achieve some measure of self-sufficiency in caring for themselves.

The most simple and direct way for individuals and governments to care for distant others is by providing them with resources to help them meet their nutritional, medical, or other needs, or by advocating for changes in local customs or laws that infringe upon some individuals' rights. Direct aid and advocacy can be uncaring, however, when they are not carried out in line with the principles listed above. While direct transfers of food, money, and other resources may be necessary after a natural disaster or to provide individuals with a safety net during hard times, these transfers should for the most part be conceived as temporary. Food programs, refuge camps, and other forms of direct aid that continue for years can promote dependency, foster corruption, or undermine the ability of individuals to care for themselves. Governments and aid organizations should

---

[10] Kari Waerness writes in this regard that 'good caring should be performed in such a way that it, as far as possible, reinforces the self-sufficiency and independence of the receiver' (1987: 211).

also constantly monitor the effects of any direct aid programs on the people and countries where they exist. If programs appear to be undermining rather than enabling the ability of individuals to care for themselves, they should be discontinued. In 1996, for example, Oxfam and twelve other humanitarian organizations pulled out of Liberia when it became evident that warring groups were using their aid to purchase arms and fund the civil war (Bell and Carens 2004: 318–19). The decision of these groups to cease operations undoubtedly contributed to the death of some individuals, but was probably the right choice from the perspective of care theory. More people would likely have died if these groups had continued to provide aid, and the people of Liberia had little chance to return to their normal lives as long as the war continued. Direct aid programs should finally always be developed in consultation with the people they are intended to help and directed toward their particular needs. Many direct food aid programs, for example, have historically been driven by the food surpluses of donor countries rather than the dietary habits and nutritional needs of hungry people, and consequently have provided food that is inappropriate or nutritionally inadequate for the individuals they were intended to help (Barrett and Maxwell 2005: 178, 192, 194).

A similar set of considerations applies to advocacy work aimed at changing local customs and laws. While human rights advocates may feel fairly certain that practices such as female genital operations are wrong, they should be careful about how they attempt to bring about social change outside their home society. Top-down or externalist approaches may achieve some nominal success in stopping uncaring practices but fail to take into account all the particularities and nuances of different societies and cultures—and hence may not be very caring in the long run. It is conceivable, for example, that human rights groups might succeed in largely abolishing the practice of female genital operations from a country only to spawn a whole generation of women who are considered unmarriageable and cast out of their communities. If rights are to be implemented in caring ways, it is imperative for human rights advocates to engage local individuals in advocating for their own human rights. The Malian activist Assitan Diallo expresses this sentiment in discussing her relations with international human rights groups:

I want them to allow me to say, 'I'm suggesting you do it this way, because these people are from my country, and I think this will be better.' Again, I'm suggesting something, not imposing it on them. That's the kind of working relationship I want. (Quoted in Williams 2000: 267)

184

Care theory, too, favors this sort of partnering relationship (Robinson 1999). By partnering with local individuals, governments and human rights groups can help to foster the protection of basic rights in context-specific and culturally sensitive ways that are more likely to yield long-term care for individuals.

A second general strategy for caring for distant others involves providing monetary support and technical assistance to foreign governments and people in order to help them develop the institutions and programs necessary to support caring activities within their countries. If distant peoples are going to be able to care adequately for themselves, they need adequate food supplies, sanitary water systems, decent and accessible housing, hospitals, schools, and other social infrastructure goods, as well as medical workers, teachers, engineers, administrators, and an effective security force. In many cases, governments may not have the monetary resources or technical expertise necessary to achieve these goals on their own. Making resources available to support these projects thus represents a second important strategy of caring for distant others.

If foreign monetary and technological aid is to contribute to the care of distant others, it, too, will have to follow the two principles listed above. Most generally, governments must be held accountable for actually using foreign aid to care for their people. As William Easterly emphasizes repeatedly in his survey of failed developmental programs: 'people respond to incentives' (Easterly 2001: xii, 143, *passim*). If government officials are not held accountable for their use of loans and grants, some are likely to use these resources for their own enrichment rather than for their people's care. Here an important point can be made about governmental responsiveness. In many cases, it is not the people of a country who are in the best position to assure that their government is responsive to their needs, but the peoples and governments of other countries and international organizations. By offering loans and foreign aid only to those governments that are likely to use them to benefit their people, and declaring that no further assistance will be offered to governments that use their resources in irresponsible ways, donor governments and international organizations can provide an important incentive for governments to respond more effectively to their people's needs. This is a hard policy since it may mean refusing to lend assistance to some already impoverished governments and peoples, but it follows from the guidelines outlined above. Providing aid to a corrupt or vicious government may be worse than a waste of resources; it may serve to prop up ruthless leaders and impede people's long-term ability to achieve a decent existence. Better, then, to pressure a corrupt government to change its ways by withholding foreign aid than to continue funding it under the false pretense of caring.[11]

In attempting to foster the technical and administrative capacities of governments, donor governments and international organizations should further target resources specifically at the development of the social infrastructure goods such as water systems, community health centers, and schools that can help people to care for themselves. Care theory recommends these goals over others for a number of reasons. First, they directly contribute to the care of individuals. Foreign aid given for more nebulous goals such as economic development or debt relief are less justifiable because they may actually do very little to help individuals to meet their needs. Second, while support for the adequate care of individuals may not be sufficient for generating jobs and economic growth, they are in most cases a necessary condition for achieving these goals and contribute to long-term labor productivity (Sen 1999: 49; Streeten 1981: viii). Where people are sick, undernourished, or have had little opportunity to develop their capabilities, it is unlikely that any economic development program will enjoy significant long-term success. Third, by targeting specific programs and projects, donor governments and international organizations can hold the recipient governments more accountable for actually using foreign aid to care for their people (Easterly 2001, 2006). It is fairly easy to assess whether a sewage system or community health center has been built and is functioning, but far more difficult to hold governments accountable for achieving general goals such as economic development that depend on many factors beyond their control. Some loans and aid will, of course, still need to be directed toward job creation and economic growth; these goals, too, fall within the purview of care theory. Yet, given the hazards involved in long-distance caring, care theory generally recommends that governments and international organizations direct the majority of their resources toward supporting infrastructure goods and programs that will directly support the care of distant peoples and bring them to a level where long-term economic development may be a more viable possibility.

[11] When possible, donor governments and international organizations might try to bypass corrupt or vicious governments in order to provide aid directly to the people in impoverished countries. As experience has shown over the past fifty years, however, it can be very difficult to prevent corrupt government officials from appropriating resources for their own purposes. Rather than providing aid to these countries, it is usually better to try to pressure these governments to change their ways by withholding aid or imposing sanctions (as discussed below) upon them.

While donor governments and international organizations might target loans and technical assistance toward particular projects, they should nonetheless allow the governments and people of these countries to determine their most pressing needs and design programs to meet them. William Easterly, Joseph Stiglitz, and others have emphasized the importance of local knowledge and control in meeting local needs (Barrett and Maxwell 2005; Easterly 2001, 2006; Stiglitz 2002). Without extensive knowledge of local customs, soil quality, weather patterns, and so forth, it is impossible to know what sorts of infrastructure development or programs will be most useful to people or how they should be designed to best serve their needs. Attentiveness, responsiveness, and respect are more generally essential to effective caring. Donor governments thus might present foreign governments and people with a menu of possible programs and projects that they are willing to support (water systems, community health centers, schools, roads, teacher training, etc.), but allow them to choose the programs and projects that they consider most important in meeting their needs, or suggest others that might similarly contribute to their ability to care for themselves. In all cases, the actual design and implementation of local projects and programs should be undertaken in collaboration with local peoples.

A third general strategy for caring for distant others involves what Robinson calls a critical ethics of caring. We should work to identify and change policies that inhibit the ability of distant peoples to care for themselves. While Robinson says very little about specific policies in this regard, Thomas Pogge offers some concrete suggestions for how international law might be changed to promote the better care of people (2002). Pogge argues that many corrupt and authoritarian governments owe their existence primarily to the laws and practices of the international community rather than to their own impoverished and disempowered populations. Western governments have provided military and foreign aid to these governments even after they have proven themselves corrupt or incompetent (Pogge 2002: 22). They have likewise shown a willingness to confer resource and borrowing privileges almost automatically upon any group who manages to seize control of the government of a country.

Any group controlling a preponderance of the means of coercion within a country is internationally recognized as the legitimate government of this country's territory and people—regardless of how this group came to power, of how it exercises power, and of the extent to which it may be supported or opposed by the population it rules. That such a group exercising effective power receives international recognition means not merely that we engage it in negotiations. It means also that we accept this group's right to act for the people it rules and, in particular, confer upon it privileges freely to borrow in the country's name (international borrowing privilege) and freely to dispose of the country's natural resources (international resource privilege). (2002: 112–13)

These international privileges not only facilitate oppressive rule but also encourage coup attempts and civil wars. It is no accident, for example, that resource rich countries such as Nigeria, Angola, and the Sudan have traditionally had some of the most corrupt and unstable governments. Since the international community has generally shown a willingness to recognize the resource and borrowing privileges of whoever is able to seize power in these countries, there is great incentive for groups to attempt to gain control of these governments and, once in power, to use the country's resources to pay off supporters and protect themselves against further coups.

Pogge proposes a rather complicated solution to this problem, calling upon the people of developing countries to write constitutions or add amendments to already existing constitutions that grant resource and borrowing privileges only to democratically elected rulers (153–66). Under this arrangement, individuals or groups who seize power illegally would have no legal rights to the resource and borrowing privileges of the country. Banks or corporations who conducted business with these illegitimate governments would do so at their own risk; if these governments collapsed, the new government would have no obligations to pay off their debts or fulfill their contracts. While this constitutional approach to resource and borrowing privileges has a number of merits, it also has some serious drawbacks. First, banks and corporations who chose to do business with corrupt governments would have an incentive to ensure that they remained in power. If these corrupt governments appeared weak or unstable, international banks and corporations might take steps to prop them up in order to secure their own business interests and the repayment of loans. Second, corrupt governments might annul the old constitution after seizing power or stage mock elections, creating confusion about the legitimacy of their rule. Banks and corporations might conduct business with the new leaders under the pretence that the old provisions no longer applied or that the corrupt government was in fact a democratically elected one. Third, and most important, the people whom Pogge's plan is intended to help are in many cases the ones who are least able to establish the sorts of constitutional amendments he favors. Where corrupt leaders are firmly in power, his plan would seem to have little prospect of success.

A simpler and perhaps more effective proposal for achieving the same goals would be to place the burden of legal recognition or non-recognition on foreign states and international organizations (Kremer and Jayachandran 2006). The UN Security Council or some similar international body might be vested with authority to assess the legitimacy of governments. Governments that came to power illegally or engaged in gross neglect of their people's rights might be dubbed 'odious,' and stripped of their international borrowing and resource privileges. The international community might then announce its refusal to recognize or enforce the terms of any bank loan made to such governments, and further pressure banks not to extend loans to them. Companies and banks that chose to do business with odious governments might likewise be subjected to fines and deprived of access to capital markets (Tamm 2004). By refusing to extend borrowing and resource privileges to odious governments, the international community would remove powerful incentives that currently exist for coups and corrupt governance in many countries, and provide some incentives for the establishment of more caring governments worldwide.

There are likely to be concerns about the possibilities for abuse under this plan. Some governments might push to have the borrowing and resource privileges of other countries revoked for self-interested reasons. Some checks might be put in place, however, to guard against such abuses. The final decision to revoke the borrowing and resource privileges of a country might, for example, be put to a vote in the United Nations General Assembly, and some sort of super-majority (e.g. a two-thirds vote in favor) might be required to pass the measure. Certain fairly well-specified conditions might further be identified as necessary for starting any proceeding against a government. Clear evidence of gross human rights abuses, a persistent pattern of government corruption and neglect of people's needs, an unauthorized seizure of government power, and a few other demonstrable actions might be specified as the only conditions under which the revocation of borrowing and resource privileges might even be considered. In these ways, concerns about the illegitimate use of these powers might be mitigated. It might further be noted that unless the international community supports these measures in practice, they are in any case unlikely to be effective.

A number of other national and international policies and laws might similarly be changed to support caring worldwide. Agricultural subsidies in Europe, the United States, Japan, and other industrialized countries have helped to undermine local subsistence agriculture in many developing countries (Barrett and Maxwell 2005: 35–6, 232–3; Lappe and Collins 1986; Mies and Shiva 1993: 231–45). By effectively supporting the dumping of cheap food into foreign markets, these subsidies have driven many local farmers out of business, increased unemployment, and in many cases contributed to hunger abroad. Eliminating these subsidies would open more opportunities for local food production and thus help many individuals in foreign countries to care for themselves without foreign assistance. International intellectual property rights agreements have likewise restricted the access of many people in poor countries to basic medicines (Birdsall, Rodrik, and Subramanian 2005; Hahnel 1998; Mies and Shiva 1993). Exempting poor countries from these agreements could greatly facilitate the survival and health of many people and contribute to their long-term health and productivity. Other suggestions for changes in international laws and policies might be further generated. The policies discussed above are offered only as examples. The main point is that caring for distant others involves more than just providing individuals with direct aid and infrastructure support; it also entails critically assessing national policies and international law in order to determine whether they hinder the ability of distant peoples to develop responsive governments and care for themselves. Writing specifically on the problem of world hunger, Frances Lappe and Joseph Collins note that what most people in developing countries need is not so much more food aid as more opportunity to feed themselves. 'Our primary responsibility... is to make certain our government's policies are not making it harder for people to end hunger for themselves' (Lappe and Collins 1986: 103). This observation might be expanded to apply to all dimensions of foreign policy, including international economic agreements. In many cases, our duty to care for distant others can be best fulfilled not by sending resources to foreign countries (although some resources are surely necessary) but instead by reforming national and international laws and policies that undermine foreign peoples' ability to care for themselves.

## 4.4. Care Theory, Just War, and Humanitarian Military Intervention

In Section 4.1 of this chapter, I outlined and defended a body of universal rights based upon the universal obligation of human beings to care for one another. In Section 4.2, I argued that these rights define a universal standard for the minimally decent treatment of human beings that should be reasonably acceptable to most people. Section 4.3 discussed three general strategies for promoting and enforcing these rights internationally. This final section addresses the justifiability within care theory of the use of military force for the sake of defending and promoting these rights.

The justifiability of military force is one of the central themes of Ruddick's *Maternal Thinking*. As noted above, Ruddick argues that care theory generally supports a nonviolent peace politics. By her account, violence breeds a number of bad consequences that should make us hesitant ever to use it. 'The effectiveness of violence is repeatedly exaggerated, while its moral, social, political, economic, psychological, and physical costs are minimized or ignored' (1989: 138). Ruddick nonetheless does acknowledge that violence may sometimes be necessary and justifiable under care theory, but does not clearly define the conditions under which military actions might be justifiably undertaken. The task here is to define these conditions more precisely.

The sole justification for the use of military force in care theory is to ensure people's physical security and support their ability to care for themselves and others. Since our own care does not morally trump the care of others, we are never justified in using military or any other form of force to take resources away from others who need them to care for themselves. It might nevertheless be morally justifiable in some cases for a group to use military force to seize excess resources from another people when the group has no other means to satisfy its basic needs.[12] Yet, for this justification to apply, the aggressor group must have no other means to satisfy their basic needs, and the group under attack must have an excess of resources that they refuse to relinquish. Even then, the use of military force would only be justifiable if it conformed to all the other conditions for the justifiable use of military force discussed below. As a practical matter, it is therefore unlikely that one people could ever justify in terms of care theory the use of military force against another people in order to seize resources from them. In practice, care theory justifies the use of military force primarily only for defensive purposes, or more precisely, to protect a people's ability to care for themselves.

Even when the aims of military force are justifiable, care theory authorizes its use only under certain conditions. First, as Ruddick argues, we

[12] St. Thomas Aquinas argues in a similar vein that one may lawfully appropriate the goods of another when necessary to meet one's own needs (*Summa Theologiae*, II-II, 66, 7; 2002: 139–40).

should use military force only as a last resort. Since caring means at the very least not harming others unless absolutely necessary, we should seek alternatives to violence whenever possible. This does not mean that we must actually try all other means before using military force, but only that all non-military options must appear futile (Brown 2002: 106). Care theory further justifies the use of military force only when it is carried out by a legitimate authority. A legitimate authority may be defined as a government or government-like body responsible for, or capable of taking responsibility for, the collective physical security and care of a people. Violent acts of resistance against an occupying force may be unjust if they do not have as their direct purpose the goal of restoring people to a condition of security and peace or are undertaken by a group that would be incapable of effectively looking after the security and care of a people if their resistance were to succeed. Care theory also endorses the principles of proportionality and discrimination in all military actions. These provisions mean that no more military force should be used than absolutely necessary to accomplish caring aims (proportionality) and every effort should be taken to avoid harming non-combatants (discrimination). These two limits on excessive violence tend to be the most controversial aspects of just war theory, but find a fairly straightforward justification in care theory. We all have a duty to care for all human beings. A central component of caring for human beings is to avoid causing them unnecessary and unwarranted pain and suffering. This duty applies importantly even to enemy combatants. While we are justified in killing enemy combatants in self-defense and in defense of our compatriots or allies, we are not justified in using excessive means against them or striking out against non-combatants. Our universal obligation to care for all people places limits on the forms of violence we can justifiably use against others. Generally recognized international rules for the humane treatment of captured enemy combatants, including prohibitions on torture, also follow from these considerations.

In general, then, care theory supports many of the well-established principles of the just war tradition. Like just war theory, it justifies the use of military violence only for the sake of securing the safety and care of people, as a last resort, when authorized by a legitimate authority, and when used proportionately and discriminately. Care theory nonetheless offers a fresh perspective on this tradition. It redefines concepts such as 'legitimate authority' in a functional way to apply to any group capable of guaranteeing peace and care to all people in a given area, and reorients the fundamental justification for war around the goal of ensuring

192

all individuals of adequate care. Perhaps most importantly, it provides an alternative justification for just war principles. Just war theory emerged in the Christian West and has no exact equivalent in other traditions (Brown 2002: 103). While most cultures have some rules that govern the conduct of war, these rules tend to be different from those of just war theory (Christopher 2004: 8–16). By rooting a form of just war theory in our obligation to care for others, care theory broadens the scope of this tradition. It demonstrates that the rules of the just war tradition are not necessarily grounded in Christian or liberal principles, but can also be justified in terms of our universal obligation to show all others at least some modicum of care.

In considering the justifiable uses of military force, a further question arises concerning its use for humanitarian purposes—specifically to protect individuals in other countries from human rights abuses. While the UN Charter clearly prohibits states from using force except for self-defense and actions authorized by the Security Council, there is a long tradition in international law supporting the morality of humanitarian military actions (Buchanan 2003b; Chesterman 2001; Franck 2003). Since 1991, governments have also increasingly defended the legitimacy of military interventions to stop gross human rights abuses (Christopher 2004; Holzgrefe and Keohane 2003; Ignatieff 2001). Care theory generally supports the justifiability of intervening into other states for humanitarian purposes, but once again only under some fairly stringent conditions.

Care theory most generally justifies the use of military force to ensure people's physical security and support their ability to care for themselves. Governments have primary responsibility for protecting and caring for the people within their jurisdictions. Yet, if the government of a country fails or refuses to protect some part of its populace from harm or actively oppresses them, then other governments and people assume responsibility for their security and might justifiably use military force to protect them. The usual objection to humanitarian military intervention is that it violates state sovereignty. Care theory, however, makes the recognition of state sovereignty conditional upon a government's willingness to care for its people. When states are unable or unwilling to care for their people, foreign states are justified in intervening to fulfill their residual obligations to care for them—but only under certain conditions.

As with military violence generally, humanitarian interventions are only justifiable as a last resort. If a government is unable to care for its people because of a lack of resources, then the international community should provide it with the resources it needs. Before resorting to

*What if this harms citizens in the process?*

military violence, the international community should likewise threaten or impose diplomatic and trade sanctions, or strip governments of loan and resource privileges, to stop human rights abuses. Military force should only be considered when all non-military options appear futile. As in other military actions, care theory also requires governments to act proportionately and discriminately in humanitarian interventions, using violence in constrained ways and only against combatants. Governments are further justified in intervening into foreign countries only when there is a reasonable chance of success.[13] Success here means not only protecting individuals from immediate threats to their survival and functioning but also returning them to their normal lives as quickly as possible. Military interventions that are likely to cause extensive damage to the social infrastructure of a country may therefore not be justifiable under care theory. While they may save the lives of some people in the short run, they may contribute to the death of tens of thousands of people in the long term from malnutrition, dehydration, and infectious diseases (Kennedy 2004, 299). Robert Keohane argues in this regard that the decision to intervene into a country should depend to some extent 'on prospects for institution-building "after intervention"' (Keohane 2003: 276). Military interventions that are undertaken without careful planning for the long-term care of the people of a country are generally unjustified. Humanitarian interventions will therefore usually look very different and employ different strategies from defensive wars against aggressor countries. The two justifications for military action are not easily interchangeable.[14]

Humanitarian military intervention is finally justified under care theory only when supported and authorized by the UN Security Council or some similar body representing the international community. Given the Security Council's refusal to endorse military intervention in places such as Kosovo in 1999, this final condition might seem overly restrictive. If

[13] This principle is often applied to just war theory generally. Yet it makes little sense to say that people are justified in defending themselves against an unjust aggressor only when they have a reasonable chance of successfully repelling the attackers. Unjust attackers are unlikely to care decently for the people they are attacking; thus people would seem to be justified in defending themselves against unjust aggressors even when the likelihood of success is small. Humanitarian interventions, however, raise different issues which make success a relevant criterion.

[14] In the Iraq war that began in 2003, the Bush administration in the United States initially justified military action on the grounds that Iraq represented a threat to the security of the United States, but then shifted to the claim that the invasion was necessary to liberate the Iraqi people from an oppressive leader. Yet the means used to invade Iraq and lack of a rebuilding plan belie the humanitarian justification.

the UN Security Council fails to take action in some case of gross human rights abuse, then surely it would seem justifiable for individual states to take action on their own. Care theory nonetheless supports international authorization for a couple of reasons (Chesterman 2001). It helps to ensure that military intervention will be used only as a last resort and in cases where governments are engaging in or tolerating what are generally agreed to be gross abuses or neglect of human rights. The very uncertainty of international approval further decreases the likelihood that groups will try to draw foreign states into their conflicts by provoking atrocities against their own people. In short, international authorization represents an important check on the use of military violence which, as Ruddick emphasizes, should be avoided whenever possible. Given the dubious justifications for and results of many past 'humanitarian' interventions, this last provision represents an important means for helping to ensure that humanitarian military interventions are carried out in line with the aims and virtues of care theory (Brown 2002: 152–9).

As distinct from the three general strategies discussed in Section 4.4, military intervention into another country is generally not morally obligatory under care theory. The different moral status of humanitarian intervention arises from the risk involved. We have an obligation to care for others only when we can do so without incurring great danger to ourselves or imperiling our long-term functioning. Because military interventions usually involve some danger to the intervening troops, they are in most cases not obligatory but supererogatory. The governments and peoples of countries would certainly be doing a great good by risking their lives—or more precisely, the lives of their troops—to stop human rights abuses in foreign countries. Yet peoples and governments have no moral obligation to undertake these actions insofar as they involve great danger to the intervening troops. Where military action stands a reasonable chance of success without greatly endangering the intervening troops, then it might be obligatory. If the international community can stop a genocide and stabilize the situation within a country by authorizing the selective bombing of certain military installations, for example, it usually ought to do so. In general, though, care theory does not recognize any duty of individuals to risk their lives for the safety and protection of distant others.[15]

---

[15] Military service in wars of self-defense raise a different set of considerations about our obligations, since presumably one's own life and the lives of one's loved ones would be threatened by the aggressor country.

## 4.5. Conclusion

All human beings depend upon other human beings to survive, develop, and function. Because we all depend upon other human beings to survive, develop, and function, we all make claims on other human beings for care. Our universal dependency on other human beings for care thus gives rise to a universal framework of human rights. We should all help other human beings to satisfy their basic biological and developmental needs and more generally to survive and function without pain and suffering since we have all called upon other human beings to help us to achieve these aims. These dictates follow from our interdependent human nature and would seem to represent the minimal requirements of any adequate human morality. Perhaps not surprisingly, then, caring for others is widely recognized around the world as a basic precept of human morality, and more generally can provide a generally acceptable standard of justice across diverse societies, cultures, and religious groups.

Caring for others in international relations may take a variety of forms. We may care for distant others by providing them with temporary emergency assistance; offering them grants, loans, and technical assistance to develop their infrastructure and public services; reforming national and international laws so that they do not undermine foreign peoples' ability to care for themselves; or using military force to protect people from unwarranted attacks from other states, their own governments, or other groups. The goal of all these activities is to support the survival, development, and functioning of individuals, and ultimately to enable people as much as possible to care for themselves.

Care theory does not provide a complete foreign policy theory. Governments will have to engage in other activities in order to maintain their national defense and security. The strategies described above nonetheless should form a core part of the foreign policy of any just government or people. The duty to care for others is not exhausted at the threshold of our homes or the borders of our countries but extends to all other human beings in the world. While we may not always be able effectively to support the adequate care of all people, we should at least do what we can to promote this goal whenever possible. Caring represents a basic morality at the heart of all human relations.

# 5

# Care Theory and Culture

A caring society depends upon more than just caring institutions and policies; it also requires a citizen body that by and large is willing to support and comply with these institutions and policies. Unless people are generally willing to support and comply with caring institutions and policies, these institutions and policies are unlikely to be implemented, or even if implemented, are unlikely to remain stable over time and function effectively.[1]

People's willingness to support and comply with caring institutions and policies, in turn, depends in large part upon their having a caring disposition. A caring disposition may be defined as having two central elements: (*a*) a broad sense of sympathy and compassion for others, meaning that one feels concern for others and desires to see their needs and suffering addressed and (*b*) a positive disposition toward caring practices themselves. Researchers have found that sympathy and compassion play a central role in motivating caring, sharing, and altruistic attitudes and behaviors (Eisenberg 1992: 44–9; Eisenberg and Fabes 1998: 733–5; Nussbaum 2001: 327–42).[2] They are not sufficient in themselves for

---

[1] Rawls discusses the problem of stability in Ch. 8 of *A Theory of Justice* ([1971] 1999: 397–449), and revises his theory of justice in *Political Liberalism* ([1993] 1996) in large part to provide a better account of stability.

[2] The terms compassion, sympathy, pity, and empathy appear in texts and common usage usually without clear distinction (Nussbaum 2001: 301). When discussing the emotions central to caring, however, care theorists have tended to distinguish between sympathy and compassion, on the one hand, and empathy, on the other hand, and have generally emphasized the importance of sympathy and compassion over empathy. They argue that sympathy and compassion connote a 'feeling with' others that respects their difference and leads to good caring while empathy involves 'putting oneself in another's place' in a manner that can be distorting, controlling, presumptuous, and paternalistic (Donovan 1996: 149; Noddings 2002: 13–14; White 2000: 113–14, 121; see, however, Meyers (1993) who argues for empathy over sympathy). Robert Solomon and Martha Nussbaum similarly emphasize the importance of sympathy and compassion in promoting caring attitudes and behaviors. They note that whereas sympathy and compassion generally connote feelings of concern for

a caring disposition, however, since a person might be broadly sympathetic and compassionate toward others but still think badly about caring activities—perhaps because he or she thinks them below his or her dignity or in some sense shameful.[3]

If people do not have a caring disposition, they may fail to see the value of caring for others or lack the motivation to establish or support caring institutions and policies. Then a caring society will have trouble taking root and maintaining itself. While some people might, of course, support and comply with caring institutions and policies strictly out of a sense of moral obligation or to avoid punishment, these grounds of support are unlikely to be stable over time. If people do not also *feel* the obligation to support caring institutions and policies, they may try to cut them back or overturn them when the opportunity presents itself.

Many care theorists suggest that human beings possess a natural sentiment of sympathy and compassion for others (Baier 1994; Donovan 1996; Luke 1996). Following Rousseau, Hume, and other natural sentiment theorists, they claim that no one 'is absolutely indifferent to the happiness and misery of others' (Hume [1751] 1983: 43 n.19). From this perspective, the moral motivation to support a caring society should already exist in most people. Even assuming that people are born with a natural sense of sympathy and compassion for others, however, these sentiments still must be cultivated if they are to exercise influence over human behavior. Contrary to Hume's hopeful pronouncement above, sympathy and compassion can be virtually extinguished in children through physical abuse and severe neglect, and even turned into their opposite (Eisenberg

others and distress at their misfortunes, empathy is a more neutral 'strategy for sharing and understanding emotions, an effort to put oneself in the other's place' (Solomon 1995: 225; Nussbaum 2001: 327–35). In this regard, a torturer might empathize with the suffering victim but only for the sake of conjuring up new and better techniques for causing pain (Nussbaum 2001: 329). Nancy Eisenberg and Richard Fabes further note that 'sympathy is an affective response that frequently stems from empathy (but can derive directly from perspective taking or other cognitive processing), and consists of feelings of sorrow or concern for the distressed or needy other,' whereas empathy can generate an 'aversive emotional reaction' that can cause a person to turn away from someone in need (1998: 702, 740). For all these reasons, I focus on sympathy and compassion rather than empathy as the emotions central to motivating caring actions. Some of the psychologists I discuss in this chapter nonetheless use the term 'empathy' to designate what I mean by compassion and sympathy: a sensitivity to the needs and suffering of others combined with a feeling that others' neediness and suffering should be addressed (Nussbaum 2001: 302). As long as one keeps in mind the general meaning of the emotion I am discussing, the use of different terms should not be too confusing.

[3] I use the terms sympathy and compassion interchangeably, although Nussbaum notes, 'If there is any difference between "sympathy" and "compassion" in contemporary usage, it is perhaps that "compassion" seems more intense and suggests a greater degree of suffering, both on the part of the afflicted person and on the part of the person having the emotion' (Nussbaum 2001: 302).

and Fabes 1998: 713). Abused or neglected children have been found to respond to the needs or suffering of other children, for example, not with sympathy or compassion but rather with contempt, anger, and even violence against them (Goleman 1995: 197–9).

While earlier chapters have focused on outlining a rational justification for our duty to care for others and describing the institutions and policies of a caring society, this chapter addresses the question of how a general disposition to care, including the emotions of sympathy and compassion and a general respect for caring itself, can be more fully developed in people. Social institutions such as those discussed in earlier chapters can play some role in this process. Martha Nussbaum notes that 'institutions teach citizens definite conceptions of basic goods, responsibility, and appropriate concern, which will inform any compassion that they learn' (Nussbaum 2001: 405). In the United States, for example, the Individuals with Disabilities Education Act helped to break down stereotypes about children with disabilities and foster compassionate understanding for them (422). More generally, where institutions and policies exist that provide support and accommodation to caring practices, individuals are more likely to recognize caring for others as a moral and social good. Alternatively, societies without caring institutions and policies may send the message to citizens that the needs of others are inconsequential or a private responsibility. Thus, 'The relationship between compassion and social institutions is and should be a two-way street: compassionate individuals construct institutions that embody what they imagine; and institutions, in turn, influence the development of compassion in individuals' (405).

Bo Rothstein and Eric Uslaner further note that social welfare programs supporting economic equality and equality of opportunity play an essential role in fostering a sense of generalized trust among people. A sense of generalized trust, in turn, encourages more individuals to engage in caring activities such as volunteer work, donating to charities, and supporting policies that provide aid to individuals in need (Rothstein 1998, 2005; Rothstein and Uslaner 2005; Uslaner 2002). Rothstein and Uslaner explain that in egalitarian societies people are more likely to perceive a common stake with others and to see themselves as part of a cooperative social system where people care about their welfare. They are therefore more likely to have a generalized sense of trust for others and engage in activities and support programs that provide care for others. While Rothstein and Uslaner's definition of generalized trust is not exactly the same as a general caring disposition, it is very close. Rothstein and Uslaner define generalized trust as 'a sense of social solidarity' and belief 'that the various groups in society have a shared fate, and that there is a responsibility to provide possibilities for those with fewer resources' (2005: 42). Individuals with a sense of generalized trust further share a number of traits in common with caring individuals including the view that the world is generally a benevolent place and a sense of efficacy in affecting events around them—as discussed below (Uslaner 2002: 23). One way, then, to encourage the development of more caring dispositions among people is to establish more public policies promoting a more equitable distribution of wealth and more equality of opportunity, such as those discussed in Chapters 2, 3, and 4. Public support for caring policies can also bring public recognition and respect to these often devalued and ignored practices. If more caring institutions and policies were implemented, more people would likely come to see caring as a public good and accept their own social dependency and the dependency of others without shame or disgust (Nussbaum 2001: 405, 421–5). In this regard, caring institutions and policies would partially generate their own support.

General social welfare programs, however, can only do so much. While these programs may be able to promote a generalized sense of trust and caring, they are likely to be established only where people are already trusting and caring. Thus, societies with low levels of trust and sympathy may find themselves in a sort of social trap: 'Social trust will not increase because massive social inequality prevails, but the public policies that could remedy this situation cannot be established precisely because there is a lack of trust' (Rothstein and Uslaner 2005: 70). In the United States, for example, Uslaner notes that levels of generalized social trust have declined since the 1960s in tandem with cuts to social welfare programs and increases in social inequality. As social programs and equality have declined, people have become less trusting, fueling more cuts in social welfare programs and more social inequality (Uslaner 2002: 160–89). Rothstein and Uslaner offer few suggestions for escaping from this vicious circle.[4] Uslaner does note, however, one important source for the development of trust outside general social and economic reforms. Generalized

[4] Rothstein and Uslaner write, 'We have a somewhat pessimistic conclusion about the political possibilities of increasing equality by enhancing universal social policies in developing and post socialist countries. Since social trust is a measure of how people evaluate the moral fabric of their society, there is little reason to believe that countries with low social trust will establish universal social programs precisely because such programs must be based on a general political understanding that the various groups in society share a common fate' (2005: 43). Rothstein does offer some suggestions for political reforms based upon the historical development of the universal welfare state in Sweden, but it is not clear that even his limited reform suggestions are transferable to other contexts (2005: 167–200).

trust grows largely out of the moralistic trust that is instilled in individuals by their parents or caregivers during childhood (Uslaner 2002: 18, 21, 26). Even if, then, it may be difficult to build trust and sympathy from the top-down through general social and economic redistribution programs, it may be possible to build it from the ground up by fostering more caring parenting practices and other cultural reforms. Indeed, as I argue below, the roots of caring attitudes in society (or the lack thereof) are deeper than our general political and economic institutions, reaching into the family, gender roles, educational system, and media. The long-term viability and stability of a caring society ultimately depends upon reforming these cultural institutions that play so vital a role in forming people's moral dispositions including their sentiments of sympathy and compassion and attitudes about caring.

Prior to the twentieth century, political philosophers regularly included discussions of education and moral development in their accounts of a just society (Crittenden 1990). Perhaps most famously, Socrates argued in the *Republic* that the realization of a just city depends upon radical reforms to society's family life, gender roles, education, and poetry. I similarly argue for reforms to family life, gender roles, education, and the media (the modern day equivalent of poetry), but suggest that less radical reforms are necessary to achieve a caring society than those suggested by Socrates. The realization of a caring society is far less demanding than the realization of Socrates' just city because the aims are more modest. A caring culture depends upon nurturing a set of minimal moral values that most people already consider good (e.g. helping others in need and helping others to develop their basic capabilities), whereas Socrates' just city depends upon cultivating a philosophical love of the truth and good. These lower aims also mean that no philosopher monarch is necessary to achieve a caring society.

My project nevertheless does confront a conundrum not unlike the one that Socrates encountered in outlining his vision of an ideal city. He argued that his just city was unlikely ever to be realized here on earth because most people are unlikely ever to assent to his cultural reforms. Even with the lower aims and less radical reforms of my project, it might still seem that few people who are not already caring would be likely to support policies designed to make our cultural institutions more supportive of caring values. Once again, then, we seem here to confront a social trap: the development of more caring society depends upon political reforms to our cultural institutions, but citizens are unlikely to support these political reforms unless they are already compassionate and caring. There seems a sort of chicken-or-egg dilemma here. Fortunately, there is a way out of it. One need not be a particularly caring person to support many of the cultural reforms I outline below. Many of these reforms are likely to generate social goods such as making people more cooperative, well adjusted, and productive, and less aggressive, antisocial, and unproductive.[5] Even a hard-hearted egoist might therefore find some merit in many of these policies, and anyone who is even minimally socially minded is likely to find some of these reforms attractive for one reason or another. We therefore do not need to await the formation of a caring citizenry to reform our cultural institutions; there are reasons for supporting these cultural reforms other than a caring concern for others. The long-run effect of these reforms is nonetheless likely to be the development of a citizen body more favorably disposed to establishing and supporting caring institutions and policies for caring reasons.

This chapter is distinct from earlier chapters in that it focuses specifically on the political culture of the United States. The analysis will be more or less relevant to people in other countries to the extent that their cultural institutions are more or less similar to those of the United States. The narrower focus here is dictated by the topic. While it is possible to outline reforms in the areas of politics, economics, and international relations that apply fairly broadly across different societies and cultures, cultural institutions are more particular and variable. Family life and child-raising practices vary quite a bit across cultures, as do aspects of gender roles, the nature of education, and the media. It is therefore necessary to focus this discussion on one particular society, and since mine is the United States, it is the subject of my discussion here. Even within the United States, there is a good deal of variation in patterns of caring among different groups and families (Collins 2000). There is nonetheless enough similarity among families and groups to identify some general

---

[5] Rothstein and Uslaner similarly highlight the benefits of a more trusting society, and thus indirectly the benefits of universal welfare programs. Particular reforms to cultural institutions are, however, likely to yield more tangible and immediate social benefits than broadly redistributive political and economic policies. The piecemeal nature of these cultural reforms also means that they can be implemented gradually and take effect over time. Rothstein and Uslaner also sometimes exaggerate the power of social traps. Not everyone need support political and economic policies, or the sorts of cultural policies I discuss below, before they can be put into place. A coalition of care advocates might push for some of these policies, and insofar as they can demonstrate the positive benefits of these policies for businesses and society generally, they might be able to get a majority of legislators to vote for them. In this regard, a fairly small group of people might be able to help society to emerge from a social trap without there already existing a broad level of trust and sympathy among the general population.

reforms that are likely to promote more caring dispositions among the majority of people.[6]

This chapter begins by surveying recent psychological research on factors that contribute to the development of caring and sharing attitudes and behaviors among people. Drawing upon this research, I outline a number of family policies (some of which have already been mentioned in earlier chapters) that can help support the development of caring dispositions among children. Section 5.3 focuses more specifically on how the gendered division of caregiving in families and society at large tends to stifle the development of caring dispositions in boys and men, and suggests polices to remedy this developmental dynamic. I then explore ways in which schools can foster more caring attitudes and behaviors in children, paying special attention to Nel Noddings's writings on caring and education. Section 5.5 explores the influence of the media, and particularly television, on caring attitudes.

The question of why people are not more caring and what can be done to make them so is obviously a large and complicated one that cannot be exhaustively addressed here. It deserves far more attention from philosophers, psychologists, educators, political scientists, sociologists, and others. This chapter represents only a beginning attempt to draw together the work of psychologists, philosophers, care theorists, and others into a synoptic account of a caring culture. The aim is to describe some of the main factors that contribute to the development of caring dispositions among people in advanced Western societies, and especially the United States, and to suggest some political policies that would likely foster more caring people. It is, however, only a beginning.

One final caveat is necessary. Much of my argument focuses on policies that are likely to encourage individuals to develop sympathy and compassion for others and engage in more pro-social or caring behaviors. It is not necessarily the case that individuals who are more sympathetic, compassionate, and caring on a personal level would necessarily support caring institutions and policies on a broad social level. However, personal sympathy, compassion, and caring do provide the moral ground for the development of a more generalized sense of caring and trust for others in society at large (Uslaner 2002: 18–21). Moreover, it seems plausible to assume

---

[6] Research seems to indicate that, if anything, the family lives and cultures of African-Americans and Latinos are more conducive to the development of caring dispositions than the traditional white, middle-class, heterosexual family (Tronto 1993: 82–5). The reforms I outline are intended both to better support families and cultures that already promote caring values, and to nudge others in the direction of more caring arrangements.

that individuals who are more sympathetic, compassionate, and caring on a personal level would on average be more likely to support caring institutions and policies in society at large, especially if efforts are made in the schools and other cultural institutions to expand their sense of sympathy and caring to individuals outside their immediate social circles.

## 5.1. The Pro-social Personality

Samuel and Pearl Oliner's book *The Altruistic Personality* (1988) provides one of the most compelling accounts of the factors that contribute to the development of caring and helping behaviors among people. The Oliners interviewed almost 700 people who either helped or did not help Jewish individuals to hide or escape from the Nazis during World War II in Nazi-occupied countries in Europe. Since helping these individuals (which included hiding them, protecting them, feeding them, and so forth) placed the rescuers and their families at considerable risk, the rescuers may be said to have engaged in a supererogatory form of caring. One usually has no moral obligation to care for others when it involves significant risk or danger to oneself or one's dependents. Surprisingly, though, most of the rescuers did not see themselves as moral heroes. In response to the question, 'Why did rescuers do it?', one Dutchman who sheltered a Jewish family for two years replied: 'I did nothing unusual; anyone would have done the same thing in my place' (Oliner and Oliner 1988: 113). Many other rescuers provided similar sorts of responses, 'saying they "had no choice" and that their behavior deserved no special attention, for it was simply an "ordinary" thing to do' (222). Based upon these responses, the Oliners concluded that helping individuals in distress was less a decision or choice made by individuals at a crucial juncture than a manifestation of an established character and moral disposition (222). The rescuers helped those in need because they were the sort of persons who did such things and could not imagine doing otherwise.[7]

Through an extensive questionnaire, interviews, and qualitative and quantitative analysis, the Oliners developed composite sketches of the personalities or moral dispositions of rescuers and nonrescuers. Nonrescuers tended to be more self-centered and mistrustful of others than rescuers, and tended to have more constricted views of the external world, looking upon others as peripheral except insofar as

[7] In her recent study of rescuers, Kristin Monroe similarly argues that rescuers acted to help Jews and others not so much by reason or choice but because they considered helping others in need as central to their characters or identities (2004).

they might be useful to them (146: 251). They generally distanced themselves from others and isolated themselves emotionally, and were more likely to hold negative stereotypes of Jews (146, 150–5, 251–2). Many of the nonrescuers also saw themselves as less personally efficacious and less capable of affecting their environment and events around them (177). Rescuers, by contrast, were more other-oriented and receptive to others' needs (161). Their worldviews tended to be inclusive, emphasizing their similarity and connection with diverse groups, and they expressed fewer negative stereotypes of Jews (175–6). Significantly more rescuers than nonrescuers accepted the importance of maintaining their attachments to other people, and rescuers also had a stronger sense of personal efficacy in influencing their environment (173, 177). Summarizing the differences between rescuers and nonrescuers, the Oliners suggested that the key to the rescuers' behavior was their positive disposition toward 'values of caring' (142–70).[8] 'What most distinguished them [rescuers] were their connections with others in relationships of commitment and care' (259). Indeed, while rescuers and nonrescuers were equally committed to values of equity and fairness, rescuers were far more likely to emphasize the importance of caring for others in need. Seventy-six percent of rescuers invoked the language of caring at least once to explain their actions:

I did it out of sympathy and kindness.

I did it out of a feeling of compassion for those who were weaker and who needed help.

When you see a need, you have to help.

Any kind of suffering must be alleviated. (164–9)

The Oliners further traced the different moral dispositions of rescuers and nonrescuers to differences in their upbringing. Rescuers more often described their early family relationships and their relationships with their mothers in particular as closer than nonrescuers did (173). Another important difference was the values that rescuers learned from their parents or other influential persons in their lives. While both rescuers

[8] Kristen Monroe also supports this conclusion, arguing that rescuers were distinguished from nonrescuers by their 'self-image as people who cared for others'. She continues: 'Because the value of caring for others was so deeply integrated into the rescuers' self-concept, it formed a self-image that was the underlying structure for their identities. This meant the needs of others were frequently deemed morally salient. This self-concept translated and transformed the rescuers' knowledge of another's need into a moral imperative requiring them to take action' (2004: 236).

and nonrescuers reported in roughly equal numbers that their parents or primary caregivers emphasized values of equity and fairness, many more rescuers said they learned generosity and caring in their homes (163–4). Rescuers also learned to be more inclusive in regard to other groups. The parents of nonrescuers taught ethical obligations to family, friends, elders, church, and country, but not to other groups. Rescuers, by contrast, reported in significantly higher percentages that their parents emphasized the duty to extend ethical consideration to all human beings (165). Finally, the parents of rescuers used far more reasoning and less physical punishment in their discipline than did the parents of nonrescuers. Nonrescuers were not only subject to more corporal punishment but also were significantly more likely to report that they were punished in arbitrary and gratuitous ways (179–80). The Oliners suggest that this factor is important because the use of reasoning rather than physical punishment in parental discipline models benevolence toward the weak and builds a sense of personal efficacy and moral responsibility in children (183).

Altogether, the Oliners found that rescuers and nonrescuers generally had different personality traits that correlated closely with different upbringings. Rescuers tended to be raised in more warm and loving homes that stressed the values of caring and inclusiveness and used reasoning as the primary mode of discipline, while nonrescuers tended to be raised by parents who were more cold and emotionally distant, rarely emphasized the importance of caring for others, and used physical punishment as the primary disciplinary method (249–51).

Recent psychological research generally confirms the Oliners' findings about the sorts of parenting activities that encourage the development of sympathy and compassion in children and pro-social or caring behaviors (Eisenberg 1992: 3, 87).[9] Parental attachments, parental modeling and teaching of caring values, and parental disciplinary techniques are all integral to the development of sympathetic, compassionate, caring, and pro-social children—that is, children, and later adults, who are more likely to engage in caring and sharing behaviors and help others in need (Eisenberg 1992: 87–110; Eisenberg and Fabes 1998).

---

[9] The next few paragraphs depend heavily on Nancy Eisenberg's summary of developmental research in *The Caring Child* (1992: 84–110) and Eisenberg and Fabes (1998). Other factors, such as genetic predisposition, also seem to play some role in determining an individual's disposition toward care. The focus here, however, is on parenting and socialization practices that most contribute to this disposition. Surveys of older literature that generally support my claims can be found in Bar-tal (1976) and Mussen and Eisenberg-Berg (1977).

The foundations of caring and pro-social behaviors are formed in children's initial attachments with their primary caregivers. John Bowlby first suggested that human infants have a basic need for a close and stable attachment with a primary caregiver, and further hypothesized that the quality of this primary attachment has long-term implications for an individual's emotional development and relationships with others (1969, 1973, 1980). Children whose parents meet their physical and emotional needs in responsive and reliable ways tend to develop a sense of trust and interdependency that provides a foundation for openness, sympathy, and compassion toward others. They come to see the people and world around them as trustworthy and dependable (Radke-Yarrow and Zahn-Waxler 1986: 212). By contrast, children whose parents do not reliably meet their needs or are excessively intrusive and controlling are more likely to view the world as hostile and insecure or maintain a sense of omnipotence that makes it difficult for them to relate to others compassionately.[10] While Bowlby's theory has been challenged and revised in a variety of ways, a substantial body of research validates some of his central theses (Fonagy 2001; Thompson 1998).[11] Children who form secure attachments with their primary caregivers—demonstrating trust that their caregivers will be there for them when needed—are generally more positively oriented and sympathetic toward others in preschool and elementary school (Elicker, Englund, and Sroufe 1992; Iannotti et al. 1992; Kestenbaum, Faber, and Sroufe 1989; Sroufe 1983; Staub 1992; Waters, Hay, and Richters 1986; Waters, Wippmann, and Sroufe 1979; Weinfield et al. 1999). Early secure attachments have also been shown to predict pro-social behaviors and sympathy among adolescents and young adults and even to predict empathy levels at age 31 (Fonagy 2001: 29–30; Grossman et al. 1999; Koester, Franz, and Weinberger 1990; Van Lange et al. 1997; Weinfield et al. 1999). By contrast, children who do not form secure attachments with their primary caregivers are more likely to become emotionally detached and mistrustful of others (Ainsworth et al. 1978). These insecurely attached children have more difficulty controlling their emotions, relating to others, feeling sympathy, and are more prone to anxiety and aggression

---

[10] Excessive or intrusive caregiving represents a perverted form of caregiving that lacks some of the essential elements of caring, such as responsiveness and respect, and ultimately aims not so much to meet the child's physical and developmental needs as to silence and control the child or perpetuate his or her sense of dependency. For a good discussion of these issues, see Nussbaum (2001: 190–200).

[11] Both Fonagy (2001) and Thompson (1998) provide surveys of the research in the field of attachment theory. Numerous other studies besides those listed in the text are referenced in their works.

(Lyons-Ruth 1996; Shaw and Vondra 1995; Shaw et al. 1997). There are, of course, numerous mediating and confounding variables that influence a child's development. Children who are more securely attached tend to make friends more easily in school, thereby reinforcing their trust and sympathy for others, while insecurely attached children usually find it more difficult to form friendships, reinforcing their sense of isolation and mistrust (Fonagy 2001: 40–41). Alternatively, insecurely attached children may develop a close relationship with a childcare worker or teacher at age 2 or 3 that mitigates the effects of an initially insecure attachment (Thompson 1998: 58–65). Early secure attachments are thus by no means determinative of a child's future social development, but they do appear to be one important factor that disposes individuals to develop more caring and pro-social attitudes and behaviors.

Bowlby initially argued that infants must attach with their own mothers in order to experience positive emotional and social development, but recent research has shown that children raised by multiple caregivers— maternal or not—can be just as securely attached, or 'if anything more so', than children raised by their own mothers (Hrdy 1999: 495; Nussbaum 2001: 187–8). Infants generally need an individual or individuals whom they can count upon to meet their basic needs and comfort and hold them if they are to develop the emotional regulation and trust necessary for caring and sympathetic relations with others.[12] However, the primary caregiver can be a mother or father, grandparent, childcare worker, or some other person, and infants can also form secure attachments with more than one caregiver at a time (Eisenberg 1992: 74–7, 100–1; Nussbaum 2001: 185–200).

Consistent with the Oliners' conclusions, researchers have also found that parental modeling and communication of caring values is important to the development of caring attitudes and behaviors (Eisenberg 1992: 88–94; Eisenberg and Fabes 1998: 715–19). Experiments show that children tend to imitate either pro-social or selfish behaviors when modeled by an adult (Eisenberg 1992: 88–9). When adults behave generously in game playing experiments, for example, children generally follow suit; when they behave selfishly, so do the children. Children whose caregivers respond sensitively to their needs likewise tend to imitate their behavior and respond sensitively to the needs of others (Bowlby 1988: 15). More generally, children whose parents engage in more pro-social behaviors,

---

[12] Attachment theorists recognize that attachments are shaped not just by objective factors but also by the infant's subjective experience, which may be influenced by temperament, biology, or other factors (Thompson 1998: 52–4).

such as performing volunteer work or working for a social justice organization, also display more pro-social behaviors than children whose parents do not engage in such activities, and children from more communally oriented cultures, such as Mexican–Americans, tend to be more compassionate and sharing than Anglo-American children (Eisenberg 1992: 89–91; Eisenberg and Fabes 1998: 707–8). In short, when children grow up in an environment where caring for others is the norm, they usually internalize a sense of responsibility for caring for others.

Teaching the importance of sharing and caring activities can also foster caring dispositions in children, but parents who teach caring values without practicing them tend to have little positive effect on their children's pro-social development (Eisenberg 1992: 92). Children can apparently see through the hypocritical and insincere pronouncements of their parents, and usually do not practice what their parents only preach. Teaching in general nonetheless can have some effect in promoting caring attitudes and behaviors, especially when they direct children to consider the emotional states of others (Eisenberg and Fabes 1998: 717–19).

Finally, researchers have found that parents who use reasoning in disciplining their children are more likely to encourage the development of caring values than those who use physical punishments (Eisenberg 1992: 95–8). Most effective in promoting sympathetic and caring behaviors are forms of discipline that call a child's attention to the harm he or she has done to others, highlight the feelings or needs of others, and encourage children to make reparations to those whom they have harmed. By contrast, power-assertive forms of discipline, including physical punishments and threats, correlate with low levels of pro-social behavior. Psychologists have suggested a number of reasons for the disparate effects of these different forms of discipline. Parents who direct their children's attention to other people's needs and feelings teach their children to take on the perspective of others and sympathize with them. Teaching children to sympathize with others, in turn, is highly effective in inducing caring behaviors (Eisenberg 1992: 44–9, 101–4). Disciplining through reasoning also communicates to children that they are in control of their lives and morally responsible for their behaviors, thus encouraging them to internalize caring values. Conversely, Nancy Eisenberg writes:

Children who are harshly punished will not be motivated to attend to what their parents say or to try to please their parents. Rather, these children will tend to be frightened in disciplinary contexts, and they will focus on their own needs rather than on those of other people. Thus, children who are frequently disciplined with

209

punitive tactics may not learn to empathize with other people, and they may learn that the primary reason for performing behaviors such as helping others is to avoid punishment. Consequently, they will not be motivated to assist others when there is no threat of punishment, and they will not internalize values related to altruism. (1992: 98)[13]

Several general conclusions follow from this discussion. The inclination to care for others appears to be more a character disposition than a choice. It is stronger in individuals whose parents raised them in ways that cultivate their sympathy and compassion than in individuals whose parents did not. Individuals can, of course, choose to act differently from their inclinations or character if they so desire. Yet the manner in which one is raised appears to have a strong influence on one's basic tendencies to care or not to care for others. Children who are raised by reliable and responsive parents who model and emphasize caring behaviors and consciously try to teach their children to think about the effects of their actions on others are more likely to be caring than those raised by unreliable, emotionally distant, self centered, and authoritarian parents.[14]

## 5.2. Family Policies for Nurturing Caring Individuals

What, then, can government do to encourage parents to raise their children in a manner more likely to foster in them the development of sympathy, compassion, and caring? The foregoing argument might seem to suggest that the best means for cultivating a more caring populace would be for government to take the care of the young into its own hands. Government childcare workers might raise children in public nurseries according to the principles outlined above so as to optimize the development of their caring attitudes and behaviors. Socrates adopted this solution in the *Republic*, arguing that traditional families should be

---

[13] Eisenberg notes, however, that 'if power assertion is used in a measured and rational way by warm, supportive parents who usually use other forms of discipline, it may not have detrimental effects on the child's prosocial development' (1992: 98).

[14] It should be noted, however, that permissiveness is not conducive to fostering caring values. Eisenberg notes that 'adults who treat the child warmly regardless of the child's behavior are not necessarily imitated, especially if the imitated prosocial behavior is costly. Perhaps children interpret such noncontingent warmth from adults as indicating that they can do whatever they please without incurring disapproval' (1992: 91). William Damon similarly argues that authoritative (but not authoritarian) parenting, marked by responsiveness, clear communication, and demands for maturity on the part of children, is most effective in fostering socially responsible children. Both permissive and authoritarian forms of parenting are less effective in achieving this aim (Damon 1988: 51–72).

abolished (at least among the guardian class) so that children could be raised in communal nurseries by professional caregivers who would foster in them the proper attitudes about justice. Nothing so drastic is necessary, however, for fostering a more caring society. In fact, Socrates' proposal for communal family arrangements might actually undermine the basic aims of a caring society. Aristotle criticized Socrates' proposal for communal childrearing on the grounds that children are likely to receive better care when raised by their parents or other loving adults, and a similar principle applies here (1995: 39–45, 1261a–1262b). If we want to raise philosophers, then communal childrearing arrangements might be appropriate, but if we want to raise sympathetic and compassionate citizens, then some form of family care is probably better.

While not all parents or parenting figures may be optimal caregivers, the vast majority do feel great love and solicitude for their children and are on average more likely to form warm and stable attachment relationships with them when given the opportunity than are government-assigned caregivers. Rather than attempting to replace parent–child relationships, the government thus might more effectively encourage the development of pro-social or caring children by instituting programs that aim to support and augment good parenting practices and compensate for poor parenting when necessary. Governments should nonetheless also remain vigilant against child abuse and severe neglect. The immediate dangers of abuse and neglect to children, and the long-term effects of these traumas on them, are usually so great that governments are well justified in removing abused or neglected children from their homes and placing them in *quality* foster-care or childcare institutions.[15]

One policy for encouraging the development of more caring and pro-social children is subsidized family leaves from work for new parents or caregivers. Subsidized family leaves were previously discussed in Chapters 2 and 3 as a means for meeting infants' basic needs and making it easier for new parents to balance the demands of work and care. Here an additional justification may be added for subsidized parental leaves. If, as suggested above, children's capacity for sympathy, compassion, and pro-social development is contingent in part upon forming a stable attachment with a primary caregiver or caregivers during the first

---

[15] The current foster care and orphanage systems in the United States is another public policy area that calls out for reform according to the principles of care theory. I cannot address this issue here, but suffice it to say that the goal of foster care should be to provide every child with a primary caregiver or caregivers who can reliably meet their physical and emotional needs in a warm and loving manner.

months of life, then it seems important that all new parents should have the opportunity to spend the first few months of their infant's life in close contact with their children. Bowlby notes that 'adequate time and a relaxed atmosphere' are necessary if parents are to care for their newborns in a manner likely to encourage the development of secure attachments, and further adds that, according to one study of new mothers, 'the most significant variable predicting differences in maternal bonding was the length of time a mother had been separated from her baby' during the baby's first six months of life (Bowlby 1988: 13, 15). One way the government thus might promote secure attachments and the development of caring dispositions in children is to mandate that all new parents are guaranteed time away from work to care for their new infants, and further offer public subsidies so that all parents have a real opportunity to take these work leaves. Research indicates that a subsidized leave of seven months (especially when coupled with flex-time policies discussed below) would be a decent minimum for forging a stable attachment (Siegel 1999: 68). Subsidies should further be set at a level that make these leaves a real possibility for all parents. Not all children will, of course, form a stable attachment relationship with their parents even under these conditions. Many other factors may intervene, including the temperament of the child and the parent's own caregiving style. Yet providing more parents with more opportunity to spend more quality time with their new infants is likely to increase the number of children who do form stable attachments—with important long-term consequences for the development of more caring children.

The government might complement family leave policies by encouraging employers to offer their workers, and especially parents with young children, the opportunity to work more flexible hours and schedules (as discussed in Chapter 3). Flexible scheduling plans include a variety of options such as offering employees the opportunity to come into work earlier in the morning and leave earlier in the afternoon, allowing them to work four 10-hour shifts during the week instead of five 8-hour days, or allowing them to work 20- or 30-hour weeks for pay and benefits proportionate to a 40-hour work week (Williams 2000: 84–100). Flexible scheduling would give parents more of an opportunity to schedule their work lives so that they could spend more time with their children and their children could spend most of their time with one or more of their primary caregivers—whether mother, father, grandparent, uncle, friend, or other—thus further promoting the formation of close and stable attachments.

The government might further provide new and expecting parents with free parenting classes or home visits from parenting instructors (Garbarino 1999: 184–7). These classes or home visits could provide new parents with much needed information about caring for their infant, their infant's development, and the likely effects of different parenting practices upon their children. Parenting instructors might talk about the importance for children of forming a secure attachment with their caregivers, the nature of appropriate attunement and responsiveness to infants, the value of modeling caring behaviors for children, and the value of noncoercive forms of discipline. One new mother who participated in a parenting class reported that 'before the program she never knew how smart babies and young children could be. Now she read to her children every night, took them to the library every Saturday, and was more confident that she could handle them without resorting to hitting' (Garbarino 1999: 185). Many well-meaning new parents may not realize what good parenting is or how important it can be to their child's growth and development—especially if they themselves were parented in less than optimal ways.

Some people may have concerns about the danger of cultural, class, or ideological biases slipping into government-sponsored parenting classes, but these dangers can be mitigated in a couple of ways. The substance of parenting classes should be restricted to basic issues relating to the care of young children such as information about nutrition, infant development, and the behavioral consequences of different parenting practices. In England, for example, the 'SureStart' program encourages parents to engage in a few basic activities, such as talking to their children, reading to them, and inviting curiosity, that helps to prepare them for success in school (Barry 2005: 52). Individuals might further be recruited from local communities to teach parenting classes in their home communities and encouraged to tailor their teachings to the particular needs and concerns of the parents there. In communities or cultures with a tradition of corporal punishment, parenting instructors might point out that arbitrary and excessive use of coercive and physical discipline usually encourages the development of traits in children that are just the opposite of what most parents desire, such as aggressiveness and a superficial regard for moral principles. In these ways, parents could be encouraged to engage in childrearing practices consistent not only with the goals of a caring society but also for the most part with their own goals for their children.

A final way in which the government might encourage the development of pro-social inclinations and behaviors in children is by ensuring access to quality childcare. The effects of childcare on young children are very controversial. Some studies have found that children who enter childcare during their early years face increased risks for aggression and social dysfunction; other studies have found no significant negative effects on children from early entry into childcare (Lamb 1998: 91–6; Maccoby and Lewis 2003). While more research needs to be done in this area, it generally appears that nonparental childcare arrangements are not harmful for most children *as long as they meet various quality measures* including low adult–child ratios, adequate levels of caregiver training, staff stability, and decent physical facilities (Blau 2001: 125–46; Helburn and Bergmann 2002: 55–85; Lamb 1998: 86–106; Scarr and Eisenberg 1993). Ideally, each child should be assigned a primary caregiver in these facilities with whom he or she might form a secure attachment. Childcare workers should likewise be trained in developmental psychology and well paid, and childcare facilities should be safe, stable, and clean. Through these arrangements, children who enter childcare during their early months will be more likely to develop secure attachments and trust in others, and children who transition into childcare after six or eight months or a year will be more likely to continue to develop in caring and pro-social ways.

Quality childcare and early education programs can further promote the development of more sympathetic and caring children in other ways. As noted in Chapter 2, early education programs have been found to have positive effects on the long-term development of poor and disadvantaged children, resulting in higher academic achievement, higher rates of employment, higher median annual earnings, more stable dwelling arrangements, and lower arrest rates (Schweinhart 2004). As such, these programs can contribute in important ways to more equal opportunity for individuals, which as Rothstein and Uslaner have shown is an important source for generating general trust and compassion for others (2005). The government could also encourage childcare centers to teach pro-social behaviors to young children. Educators and psychologists have developed a number of social emotional learning and empathy training programs that have proven highly effective in enhancing the sympathy and pro-social behaviors of young children and reducing aggression and other antisocial behaviors (Cohen 2001; Eisenberg 1992: 101–4; Eisenberg and Fabes 1998: 727–31). These programs typically teach children to identify their different emotions, to take the perspective of other people and think about their feelings, and to cooperate with others to achieve common goals (Feshbach 1982; Feshbach and Feshbach 1986). Many of these programs have been developed for elementary school age children or older, but at least some exist for children as young as 3- or 4-years old (Shure and Glaser 2001). Intervention strategies also exist for identifying insecurely attached children and helping them to develop trust and sympathy for others (Garbarino 1999: 187–91). As a condition of receiving public subsidies, governments might require childcare centers to implement one or another of these programs in order to help children further develop their sympathy and compassion for others.

In sum, it is neither necessary nor desirable for governments to assume direct responsibility for childrearing. The development of more compassionate and caring children can be better encouraged by providing more support and training to parents so that they can spend more time with their children and raise them in more pro-social ways; and by supporting quality childcare centers that can foster and teach sympathy and emotional intelligence. These policies may not succeed in fostering caring dispositions among all children, but they are likely to succeed with many of them. The education system (discussed below) can further help in this process and expand children's sympathy and compassion beyond their immediate social circles.

Absent from this discussion of pro-social childrearing has been any mention of a number of pro-family, and specifically pro-heterosexual marriage, policies that have been touted in recent years as solutions to many of society's problems. William Galston, David Blankenhorn, David Popenoe, Barbara Dafoe Whitehead, and others have argued that children's healthy development depends upon supporting and promoting the married, two-parent, heterosexual family, and to this end have endorsed policies that eliminate no-fault divorce and discourage out of wedlock births (Blankenhorn 1995; Etzioni 1993; Galston 1995; Popenoe 1996; Whitehead 1993). Blankenhorn and Popenoe further maintain that the health of families and children requires that we reject the egalitarian family model where men and women share breadwinner and childcare tasks, and recommit ourselves to the gendered division of labor where men are breadwinners and women are caregivers.

There is at least some evidence to support the argument for the importance of two-parent families. Children who grow up in two-parent families generally suffer fewer emotional and behavioral problems, perform better in school, and are less likely to engage in criminal behavior than children from single-parent families. Many of the problems associated with single parenthood, however, can be attributed to the lower incomes of single-parent families in comparison with two-parent families, and can be addressed through policies that guarantee all parents a decent income (Streuning 2002: xvi–xvii, 70–6). Other forms of support services such as subsidized parenting leaves, flex-time policies, quality childcare, health care, and a decent education for all would further help single parents to provide their children with the care they need to develop their basic capabilities and caring dispositions. Single parenting, then, need not be bad for children if supported through adequate social policies. Conversely, while children obviously benefit from growing up in a relatively happy and healthy two-parent family, the same is not necessarily true of children who grow up in homes marked by animosity and fighting (Berkowitz 1993: 188–9; Geen 2001: 92–3; Streuning 2002: 69). In fact, given what we know about parental modeling, contentious or abusive marriages might actually impede the development of sympathy and caring among children. Pro-marriage policies that encourage the traditional segregation of breadwinning and caregiving tasks are also likely to hinder the development of caring attitudes among boys and men—for reasons to be discussed in Section 5.3.[16] Many pro-marriage policies therefore do not seem especially useful in promoting caring and pro-social attitudes and behaviors, and some may actually be counterproductive to this aim. There are, of course, other religious, moral, and demographic reasons why a society might choose to promote marriage. As long as such policies do not negatively impact the ability of individuals to give and receive care, care theory is indifferent or neutral toward them. However, if the goal is to encourage the development of more caring children, there appears little to be gained, and perhaps much to be lost, by attempting to shore up marriages through measures that restrict divorces or direct men and women back into traditional gender roles.

## 5.3. Caring, Gender, and the Family

While more public support and training for parents and subsidized quality childcare arrangements would be important steps toward encouraging more caring dispositions and behaviors, the effectiveness of these reforms might be limited as long as care work continues to be organized along gender lines. In the United States and most other countries, women

[16] Streuning similarly notes that gender-based parenting is likely to undermine Popenoe's and Blankenhorn's stated goal of strengthening ties between fathers and children. 'Research suggests that the best way to foster strong ties between fathers and children is to encourage the father's involvement in infant and childcare' (Streuning 2002: 100).

perform the vast majority of care work, assuming primary responsibility in particular for the care of children. In her classic work *The Reproduction of Mothering* (1978), Nancy Chodorow argues that the gendered distribution of care work has profound implications for the psychological development of boys and girls, and ultimately for cultural attitudes about caring. 'Girls and boys develop different relational capacities and senses of self as a result of growing up in a family in which women mother' (Chodorow 1978: 173).

According to Chodorow, in the earliest, or preoedipal, period of an infant's life, mothers tend to experience and treat their daughters and sons differently. Women view their daughters as like themselves, prolong their close attachment to them, and give them less leeway for separateness and individuation (99–104). Consequently, girls tend to develop their sense of identity in close relation to their mothers and tend to have difficulty differentiating themselves from them. By contrast, mothers experience their sons as male opposites, push them more quickly out of their preoedipal attachment, and more readily encourage their differentiation and individuation (104–8). Boys thus curtail their primary love attachment with their mothers, and construct more rigid ego boundaries in forming their identities.

These early developmental tendencies are reinforced during the Oedipal period. During this period, Chodorow argues that children develop sexualized relations to their parents not because of innate libidinal drives but rather because parents tend to sexualize their relationships with their children and enforce traditional gender norms—flirting, for example, with the children of the opposite sex and generally encouraging gender appropriate behaviors (111–29). Boys respond by identifying with their fathers and further distancing themselves from their mothers. Girls, by contrast, add their fathers to their already close attachment to their mothers. The main importance of the Oedipus complex, according to Chodorow, is not so much the development of different sexual identities as 'the constitution of different forms of "relational potential" in people of different genders' (166):

From the retention of preoedipal attachments to their mother, growing girls come to define and experience themselves as continuous with others; their experience of self contains more flexible and permeable ego boundaries. Boys come to define themselves as more separate and distinct, with a greater sense of rigid ego boundaries and differentiation. The basic feminine sense of self is connected to the world, the basic masculine sense of self is separate. (169)

217

The fact that women perform the majority of primary caregiving work in our society thus has profound consequences for the development of different caring and relational capacities in girls and boys. From an early age, girls learn to relate to others and the world around them in and through relationships, while boys do so by forming a more sharply defined and closely guarded sense of self.

These dynamics carry over into the development of gender identity in later childhood and early adolescence. A girl's gender role learning and gender identification are continuous with her early identification with her mother. She learns to model her behavior after her mother and other mothering figures who are close to her. A boy's development is more complicated because he must shift his attachment away from his primary caregiver—at least insofar as his primary caregiver is his mother—to achieve his expected gender identification: 'A boy, in order to feel himself adequately masculine, must distinguish and differentiate himself from others in a way that a girl need not—must categorize himself as someone apart' (174). Boys' gender role learning is further made difficult by the general absence of fathers or adult male role models in their lives (176–7). Because girls are continually mentored by their mothers and other women, they develop particular and nuanced understandings (and sometimes insight into the contradictions) of gender roles. Boys, however, often must learn the masculine role in the absence of a close, continual personal relationship with their fathers or other adult male role models. As a result, they frequently resort to cultural norms, popular representations of masculinity, rigid role definitions, and peer opinions to define their gender identity. Above all, boys define themselves in opposition to women.

Dependence on his mother, attachment to her, and identification with her represent that which is not masculine; a boy must reject dependence and deny attachment and identification. Masculine gender role training becomes much more rigid than feminine. A boy represses those qualities he takes to be feminine inside himself, and rejects and devalues women and whatever he considers to be feminine in the social world. (181)

Since caring is associated with the feminine in most societies, boys generally repress their capacities for caring, sympathy, and relationship in forging their identities. To be a man means to be self-sufficient and independent. A caring man is a contradiction in terms, or at least a highly ambiguous figure.

Chodorow's theory goes a good way toward explaining the general devaluation of caring in American culture and many other cultures as well. Boys grow up denying and repressing relations and connection with others. They come increasingly to see caring as a threat to their identity and inappropriate except perhaps in the most intimate of relations, where they feel they can show themselves to be vulnerable. The external world or public realm is viewed as a state of nature—dangerous and threatening—where strict rules must be established to mediate relationships and protect individual autonomy. Caring practices and values are seen as largely out of place in this world, and segregated into the private realm where they are associated with the feminine. Since men have historically held the majority of power in society, their disdain for caring has generally defined the public culture. Government is conceived as an impartial arbitrator of disputes rather than a supporter of caring. The 'nanny state' is held up for particular scorn as the very opposite of what a good government should be (Folbre 2001: 84–108).

Chodorow's thesis has been criticized on a number of different grounds. Leslie Brody notes, for example, that same- and opposite-sex relationships within the family are not stable, but shift as a function of who is present in the family (1999: 153). When fathers are present, mothers show more affection toward their sons, while fathers become more distant toward their sons when mothers are present. Parent–child relationships may also vary as a function of the family's composition, including the number of children in a family, the sex of the children, marital status, and marital quality (154–5). In general, Brody argues that 'Chodorow and other feminist psychoanalytic theorists generalize too broadly across all types of families . . . [and] also inappropriately generalize from Western family life to family life in other cultures' (155). Brody offers these observations, however, more as amendments to Chodorow's thesis than as direct challenges to it. She argues that new research generally supports Chodorow's thesis about gender-differentiated interactions between parents and their children (at least in Western cultures) and their effects on children's attitudes about care and relationships, and especially emphasizes the important effects that fathers who engage in direct childcare can have on the emotional development of children (148, 153, 169, 177–97).[17]

---

[17] Brody further argues that 'gender-differentiated patterns of interaction between parents and their young children may have more to do with gender differences in infant temperament and with cultural gender stereotypes than with patterns of same-sex identification in the family' (1999: 148). Subtle differences in infant boys' and girls' sociability, activity levels,

Patricia Hill Collins (2000) further argues that Chodorow inappropriately generalizes not only across cultures but also within Western culture. By her account, Chodorow's description of mothering reflects primarily the experience of middle-class white families. In African-American communities, women often rely upon extended kin networks and informal communal childcare arrangements to raise children. As a result, many African-American children develop a more communal identity, and there exists a more generalized 'ethic of care' in African-American communities than in white ones (Collins 2000: 189–92, 262–6).

Collins's criticism is important in drawing attention to the ways in which different family and community arrangements can impact attitudes about caring. Research has found that individuals from more communally oriented cultures, including African-Americans and Mexican-Americans, tend to be more generally sympathetic and caring (Eisenberg and Fabes 1998: 707–8; Tronto 1993: 82–5). Nonetheless, Collins's argument does not wholly undermine Chodorow's claims. As long as the majority of childrearing is performed by women, one would expect that some of the developmental dynamics described by Chodorow would still apply in African-American communities.[18] The communal caring arrangements of African-Americans may foster a more communal care ethic, but since most of the primary caring is still performed by women, girls are still more likely to develop their gender identities in relation to their primary caregivers and to be more sympathetic and caring, while boys are likely to develop their identities in opposition to their primary caregivers and to distance themselves from caring values. Collins herself describes some of the interesting implications of this dynamic. Black men may glorify the 'superstrong Black mother' but are reluctant to assume primary caretaking responsibilities themselves (2000: 174). Although they appear to be more open on average than white men to affirming the importance of caring, they still show aversions to engaging in care work and tend to idealize women as caregivers.

language abilities, and self-regulation appear to have some effect on parental responsiveness. Brody nonetheless still contends that the sex of the primary parental caregiver has important effects on children's emotional development. Regarding cultural gender stereotypes, I would further note that, although Chodorow does not emphasize this point, it seems to be implicit to her theory.

[18] Chodorow writes: 'I have yet to come across any woman patient, or any narrative (fictional, autobiographical, biographical, or poetic) written from the daughter's point of view—among patients or writers of whatever sexual orientation and from whatever cultural group—for whom in the broadest sense we could say that "love" for a daughter's mother was not central' (1994: 82).

Chodorow's theory has also been challenged on empirical grounds. Chodorow's thesis seems to predict that women should on average be more likely to embrace caring values and to engage in pro-social behaviors than men. Research findings, however, are not so clear-cut. Some research does support certain aspects of Chodorow's thesis. Numerous studies show, for example, that boys whose fathers engage in caregiving show a greater capacity for sympathy and compassion, have more flexible attitudes about gender roles, are better able to express feelings of vulnerability and sadness, and are generally more caring toward others (Brody 1999: 177–97; Carlson 1984; Duindam and Spruijt 2002; Hardesty, Wenk, and Morgan 1995; Pollack 1998: 119–120; Williams, Radin, and Allegro 1992). These studies appear to support Chodorow's claim that the gendered division of labor affects individuals' moral development, and especially her claim that boys who grow up in close relation with their fathers or other male caregivers will tend to be more open to caring.[19]

Studies that have directly tested men's and women's moral orientations, however, have found that girls and women are on average only slightly more likely than boys and men to embrace caring values and engage in pro-social behaviors (Eisenberg 1992: 39–40; Eisenberg and Fabes 1998: 252–5; Jaffee and Hyde 2000). While these findings might seem to discredit Chodorow's argument, they are not as damning as they might initially appear. Chodorow nowhere suggests that the gendered division of labor is the only important factor in the development of caring or pro-social behaviors. As noted above, many other factors are also important in this process, including the quality of a child's attachment to his or her primary caregivers, parental modeling and teaching of caring behaviors, and the primary mode of parental discipline. It seems likely (and wholly consistent with Chodorow's thesis) that boys and men raised in caring homes would be as caring or more so than girls and women raised in cold and authoritarian homes. Unless these factors can be identified and held constant—as they almost never are—then crude tests of whether women or men express more caring attitudes tell us very little about the effects of gender on the development of moral dispositions. In fact, given that existing studies generally have not attempted to hold constant for different home environments, it seems significant that studies have found that girls and women are on average slightly

[19] Other factors also affect the influence of fathers' caring on children, such as the degree to which fathers practice and teach values that support traditional gender roles (Williams, Radin, and Allegro 1992).

more likely to express caring values and pro-social orientations than boys and men. Even without holding constant for all the other important factors that might determine whether a person is positively oriented toward caring, gender seems to matter somewhat. Nothing certain can be said, however, until more nuanced studies are performed. The more particular research that does exist—focusing on the effects of male care-giving on boys—nonetheless does support at least this part of Chodorow's thesis.

Toward the end of *The Reproduction of Mothering*, Chodorow suggests that the key to a more caring society lies in more equal parenting arrange-ments. If parents were equally to share in the primary care of infants and young children, children would develop their sense of self in relation to both parents. As a result, 'masculinity would not become tied to denial of dependence and devaluation of women', which in turn 'would reduce men's need to guard their masculinity and their control of social and cul-tural spheres' (Chodorow 1978: 218). Additionally, more equal parenting would help to undermine one of the more pernicious aspects of American culture's definition of masculinity: the notion that caring and nurturing are unmanly (Pollack 1998: 113–44). Chodorow's proposal seems sensible enough, especially since there is empirical evidence to support the claim that boys raised in close proximity to their fathers tend to be more caring. However, Chodorow fails to offer any policy suggestions for encouraging the development of more equal parenting or caregiving arrangements. Without some such encouragement, it is unlikely that equal parenting will be widely adopted, since individuals raised in families with gendered parenting practices may find it difficult to see the value in more egalitarian arrangements. Men may have little interest in caring for infants and may feel emasculated by doing so. Women may derive special psychic satisfaction from mothering. Chodorow offers no solutions for breaking out of this cycle of gender reproduction and nudging people toward more egalitarian caring practices.

In a new preface to the second edition of *The Reproduction of Mothering* (1999), Chodorow further backs away from her earlier proposal. 'If you take seriously that psychological subjectivity from within... is central to a meaningful life, then you cannot also legislate subjectivity from without or advocate a solution based on a theory of political equality and a conception of women's and children's best interests that ignores this subjectivity' (1999: xv). Chodorow's point is that women's subjective desire to mother ought to be respected even if it is forged out of and reproduces unequal parenting practices or a sexist culture.

Mothering is not simply another socially created unequal role that can be challenged, like the glass ceiling and discriminatory practices that keep women from achieving in the educational, economic, and political worlds. Accordingly, a feminist recognition of the centrality of the realm of psychological reality would not have singled out a demand for equal parenting as a social goal—a goal that not only ignored many women's identities, wishes, and desires but that was also easily transformed into a claim for father's rights. (xvi)

Chodorow now recommends 'institutional and political supports' that would help 'mothers to mother their children and have a full life', but otherwise refrains from offering any suggestions that might encourage parents to consider changing the traditional distribution of caregiving work (Chodorow 1999: xvi–xvii).

Chodorow's concerns are important in a country that values individual freedom and choice. Since most people in the United States consider personal freedom to be an important good, it would be inappropriate for the government to legislate parenting arrangements in a way that discounted individual preferences and beliefs. Yet, if the government does nothing to address the gendered division of labor, gender stereotypes are likely to remain largely intact, and with them, the tendency for men to devalue caring. The solution to this problem lies in identifying policies that can nudge men and women in the direction of more egalitarian caregiving while still respecting their subjective preferences. Slight modifications to some of the policies discussed in Section 5.2 might go some way toward achieving this aim.

As a first step, the government might take steps to encourage more men to take family leaves from work in order to assume primary care for infants. Janet Gornick and Marcia Meyers identify three strategies for promoting this goal (2003: 134–9). Most fundamentally, men should be offered the opportunity to take subsidized family leaves on a use-or-lose basis. After the birth or adoption of an infant, one parent might be offered a period of subsidized leave from work (e.g. seven months), and then the other parent might be offered an equal period of subsidized leave. The subsidized leaves would be nontransferable from one parent to the other, so if a father chose not to take the parental leave, the benefit would be lost. High wage replacement during family leaves is also important for encouraging men to take parenting leaves. Since men tend to have higher wages than women, there is a greater disincentive for them to take family leaves when subsidies are low. Finally, a public education campaign emphasizing the benefits of male parenting might help to reduce some of

haven't found this to be true

their resistance to take parenting leaves. While motherhood tends to be valorized in American culture, fatherhood generally is not.

Even with these policies in place, not all men would take advantage of parenting leaves, or take the full extent of their possible leave time. In Sweden, for example, where generous parental leaves exist for both parents, men on average tend to take little leave time from work (Alstott 2004: 112). The reluctance of men to take parenting leaves is not, however, a reason to not offer them (Gardiner 1997: 160). Cultural changes take time. If the steps outlined above were followed, one would expect that at least some men would take at least some time off from work to care for their infants, and over time more men would likely become more directly involved in raising their children. This policy would not greatly interfere in the emotional lives or subjective preferences of individuals, since fathers (or mothers) could simply refuse to take a work leave if they did not want to assume direct care for their children. Those men who did take the leave, however, would contribute to the development of a more caring society in several ways. First, they would be directly involved in parenting their children from a young age which would help boys, in particular, to develop a sense of identity in relation to their fathers and likely become more open to caring. Girls might also benefit from this arrangement by developing a stronger sense of independence from a young age (Brody 1999: 177–8). Carol Gilligan notes that because girls generally develop their identities in close relation to their mothers, they often have difficulty asserting themselves in relationships and recognizing care of self as a valid concern (Gilligan 1982: 128–74). As a result, they sometimes take on an undue share of the care of others even when men could easily do so. By offering girls more chance to develop their identities apart from their mothers or mothering figures, more equal parenting arrangements might make them less likely to assume the role of self-sacrificing caregivers and, in the long run, more likely to demand that men take a more equal share in caring for their own children.

If more fathers were directly involved in parenting, the cultural stereotype of caring as a feminine activity would also begin to dissipate, and men might become more willing to express caring values, perform caring tasks, and recognize caring as an important public function. Caring would then not seem so threatening to their sense of masculinity. Indeed, research has found that fathers who take a direct role in caring for children tend to become more nurturing, affectionate, and emotionally expressive (Brody 1999: 185, 222–3; Pollack 1998: 133). Finally, if more boys and men became more accepting and supportive of caring values and behaviors, more girls and women would likely feel more comfortable supporting and expressing these values and behaviors as well. At present, at least some women may distance themselves from care and compassion for fear of being stigmatized by gender stereotypes.

Another important measure for encouraging more equal parenting arrangements is the flexible work policies discussed in Section 5.2. The current organization of work in the United States strongly encourages an asymmetrical division of productive and reproductive work (Williams 2000). Many couples opt, if possible, to have one parent stay home with the children while the other engages in remunerative labor not necessarily because they consider this arrangement to be the optimal way of organizing their emotional and family lives, but because most jobs demand a full-time commitment from their employees that leaves little time for childcare. One must either work or care under these arrangements, but rarely can a person do both well (or sometimes at all). If the government encouraged employers to offer their employees, or at least new parents, flexible work schedules, those parents who desired to engage in more equal parenting arrangements would have more of an opportunity to do so. Couples could more easily arrange their schedules so that each parent could play a more equal part in caring for their child. One parent might choose to cut back his work schedule to 30 hours per week, while the other might work four 10-hour days. One or the other parent could then almost always be at home to care for the child.

These first two policies would encourage more equal parenting relationships in traditional two-parent families, but would do little to affect the gender development of children in single-parent (usually single mother) homes. A more broadly based measure for breaking down the gendered division of caregiving and cultural gender stereotypes, and providing all children with more male adult caregiving role models, would involve actively recruiting more men into childcare work and primary education. At present in the United States, ninety-eight percent of preschool and kindergarten teachers, ninety-five percent of childcare workers, and ninety-one percent of elementary school teachers are female (National Education Association 2003: 91; U.S. Census Bureau 2005: 402–3). Most children therefore encounter the same gendered division of care work outside the home that they experience within their homes. In order to help break down this gendered division of caring and fashion a more caring culture, the government might make concerted efforts to recruit more men into childcare and elementary education, initiating something like an affirmative action policy for men in these fields. An advertising campaign that recast childcare and elementary education as a civic responsibility might encourage some young men to apply for jobs in this field. The government might also offer some sort of tax incentives or subsidy to childcare and early education centers that recruited and trained more men for this work. All of this would be easier, of course, if childcare workers and elementary school teachers were better paid—as suggested in Chapter 3. While some people might find strange or even amusing the idea of an affirmative action campaign designed to recruit men into childcare and elementary education, this reaction merely serves to show just how deeply devalued caring is in many societies. As Nel Noddings points out, hardly anyone blinks an eye at programs designed to recruit more women into math and science, but no one seems to worry that young men lag behind 'in preparation for elementary education, nursing, early childhood education, or full-time parenting' (Noddings 2002: 46–7). The reason for this disparity seems to be our lack of respect for the caring professions. If a campaign were undertaken to recruit more men into childcare and elementary education, and if it were successful, more children would have the opportunity to develop their gender identities in relation to both male and female care-giving figures, and caregiving would be further affirmed as both a male and female activity.

In sum, government might encourage positive changes in the current gendered division of care work and gender stereotypes, and thereby promote more caring and pro-social attitudes and behaviors among children, by providing enticements and opportunities for more men to engage in care-giving activities both inside and outside the home. If men took a greater part in caring for children, boys would grow up to be less fearful or disdainful of caring, and people would be more likely to see caring as a valuable human, as opposed to distinctively feminine, activity. Girls would also likely develop a stronger sense of independence and be less likely to behave as selfless caregivers, thus further forcing men to take on more of the caregiving work of society. None of the policies outlined here are particularly intrusive into people's subjective or family lives, but all provide subtle incentives toward long-term cultural changes in attitudes about caring.

## 5.4. Educating for Caring

After the family and early childcare, the education system is the most important influence on children's development. As argued in Chapter 2, the primary purpose of a caring educational system should be to help all children to develop their basic emotional, imaginative, linguistic, reasoning, social, reading, writing, and math capabilities so that they can function successfully in society. Yet the educational system can also play an important role in developing the sorts of caring attitudes and pro-social behaviors necessary to support a caring society.

Nel Noddings has written most extensively on the nature of a caring education (Noddings 1984, 1992, 2002, 2003; see also Johnston 2006). 'The main aim of education', according to Noddings, 'should be to produce competent, caring, loving, and lovable people' (1992: 174). To accomplish this goal, she proposes three general reforms to the current educational practices in the United States. First, she suggests that classrooms should be made more caring places (1984: 175–97, 1992: 21–7). Teachers should be encouraged to model caring behaviors for students and exhort students to be caring toward others. Even more importantly in her estimation, teachers should practice care toward their students by designing assignments to respond to student interests and tastes. Rather than forcing students to struggle through works of classical literature, for example, they might be offered the opportunity to read contemporary books that more directly relate to their lives (2002: 294–5). Students should also be encouraged to raise and address questions in the classroom that are important to them. Most generally, Noddings calls for reflection on all classroom routines, including the use of seating charts, homework, grades, and so on, to discern whether they demonstrate care toward students (1992: 174–5, 2003: 256–8).[20]

Noddings's second general reform involves loosening curriculum requirements to better accommodate and develop the diverse interests and talents of students. Noddings recognizes that there are some things that all children must learn, such as reading, writing, communicating, basic math, and so on, and recommends that students should be required to achieve mastery in these areas. But at least in middle school and high school, she argues that many of the current curriculum requirements should be dropped, and students should be allowed to take classes that they find interesting and relevant to their life goals, such as classes in mechanics, business, art, music, computers, or other fields (2003: 205–9). Noddings questions the wisdom of requiring all students to take courses in algebra and geometry that have little relevance to most students' life goals

---

[20] Noddings also calls for more continuity in education, including keeping teachers with the same students for several years and keeping classes of students together as much as possible (1992: 62–73).

and drive some students away from school altogether. Students interested in careers in science, math, or engineering should be encouraged to take these classes, but others might take music, humanities, vocational, or other courses better suited to their interests and abilities.

Noddings's third reform involves overhauling the organization and content of the curriculum. Rather than organizing the curriculum into discrete academic disciplines, she proposes organizing it around domains of caring: 'care of self, care for intimate others, care for associates and distant others, for nonhuman life, for the human-made environment of objects and instruments, and for ideas' (1992: 47, 74–172). Ideally, she suggests that these seven domains would subsume the current liberal arts curriculum, but 'in the interest of compromise and practicality', she settles for recommending that the secondary school curriculum should be 'divided equally between the subjects as we now know them and courses devoted to themes of care' (1992: 70). In her plan, many of the isolated subjects in the current curriculum would be integrated under one or more of these domains of care. The care of self course, for example, would include elements from physical education, home economics, nutrition, drug education, sex education, and health. The care for nonhuman life course would include elements from science, math, reading, history, and ethics. These courses would further place new emphasis on education for home and private life. Students would study 'sex education, pregnancy, birth, motherhood and fatherhood, child development, home design and aesthetics, the care of nonhuman living things, nutrition, meal planning and cooking, care of those with special needs (including the elderly), home repair and safety, budgeting and consumer knowledge, moral education, exercise and recreation' (2002: 297; 2003: 95–194). Through these courses, students would be prepared for the activities of private life just as they are currently trained for public and professional life.

Noddings outlines one compelling vision for an educational system based upon care ethics. My approach departs from hers, however, in two fundamental ways. Many of Noddings's reforms focus on making schools more caring places by organizing them to be more attentive and responsive to student interests and preferences. My approach focuses on making schools more adept at fostering the development of students' basic capabilities, including their emotional capabilities for sympathy, compassion, and caring.[21] There may be some overlap between Noddings's goals and

[21] Once again, I am focusing here on how schools can contribute to the development of children's emotional capabilities, and as such do not discuss in any detailed way how schools might also better help students to develop their motor skills, imagination, reason, writing,

228

my own, but they are not necessarily the same. Martha Nussbaum, to provide only one example, makes a strong case for the importance of classical literature—Aeschylus, Sophocles, Emily Bronte, Richard Wright—for fostering sympathy and compassion in children (2001: 401–54). By her estimation, the works of these authors are important precisely because they draw students away from their everyday interests and challenge them to enlarge their sympathy and compassion for human beings in general. My own view is more in line with Nussbaum's than Nodding's argument. If students are to develop a general sense of sympathy and compassion, schools probably ought not to cater to their desires and interests on many subjects. They should instead aim to enlarge students' understanding of the human condition by asking them to study the problems and concerns of individuals who are not like them.

My approach to a caring education also has more limited aims than Noddings's. Noddings outlines an educational plan that makes 'the maintenance and enhancement of caring... the primary aim of education' (1984: 174). In other words, she argues that education should serve primarily to produce caring students. I agree that caring is an important value that the educational system should aim to cultivate. Yet schools should not necessarily subsume all other values to this one aim. There are many other legitimate values and aims that people may wish to promote through their educational systems such as a broad understanding of history or science. As such, I suggest that the teaching of caring should assume an integral place in education, but (as distinct from Noddings's approach) should not necessarily dominate it. The goal of education should be to foster the basic capabilities of children and promote more caring attitudes and behaviors but not necessarily to produce students who regard caring as their highest aim.

Some of Noddings's proposals for classroom teaching are nonetheless still relevant even given my more limited aims. Teachers can play an important role in encouraging caring and pro-social behaviors by modeling these behaviors for students, setting pro-social expectations and rules in the classroom, verbalizing the importance of caring for others, reinforcing pro-social behaviors, and using reasoning rather than threats or force whenever possible to discipline students (Eisenberg 1992: 112–22; Oliner 1985–6). While it might be assumed that most teachers already engage in these sorts of behaviors, observational studies have found that many

and other capabilities. The development of all these capabilities is nonetheless important under care theory, and other reforms would likely be necessary to cultivate these other capabilities.

teachers rarely reinforce or encourage children's pro-social behaviors and that pro-social behaviors are fairly rare in many classrooms (Eisenberg and Fabes 1998: 727). Teacher trainings should emphasize the importance of pro-social teaching, and schools should encourage teachers to promote pro-social attitudes and behaviors in the classroom.

Along these same lines, schools should incorporate social emotional learning or empathy training into their curricula. Literally hundreds of social emotional learning programs have already been developed (Cohen 2001: 5). One important component of many of these programs is co-operative learning (Johnson, Johnson, and Holubec 1991; Slavin 1990). Cooperative learning generally involves placing students in small groups and assigning them interactive and largely self-monitoring activities. Groups might be organized according to achievement levels, so that more advanced students can work on more difficult materials while less advanced students can concentrate on mastering more basic materials, or they can be organized heterogeneously so that more advanced students mentor less advanced ones. In any case, cooperative learning makes caring about other students' learning an explicit classroom goal. It conveys a message to students quite different from that of traditional classroom settings that we are all responsible for the needs and development of others and dependent upon them to accomplish our tasks. Research has shown that cooperative learning is effective not only in promoting more cooperative behaviors, more acceptance of others, and more pro-social behaviors, but also in improving cognitive and academic capabilities (Johnson, Johnson, and Holubec 1991; Slavin 1990).

Cooperative learning represents only one aspect of social emotional learning. One social emotional learning program, the Child Development Program (CDP), combines cooperative learning with several other techniques for fostering sympathy and compassion in children (Dasho, Lewis, and Watson 2001). This program includes classroom community-building exercises that address students' need for attachment and belonging, assignments that offer students an opportunity to help one another, and utilizes reason-based or inductive discipline in the classroom. The CDP programs have proven effective in promoting a number of pro-social attitudes and feelings including conflict resolution skills, willingness to compromise, concern for others, trust, and altruistic behavior (Dasho, Lewis, and Watson 2001: 104).

Other school-based programs focus more specifically on empathy training and emotional literacy (see, e.g., Kusche and Greenberg 2001). Empathy training programs teach children to recognize the feelings of others, imagine themselves in another's place, and communicate effectively (Eisenberg 1992: 101–4, 115–7; Feshbach 1982; Feshbach and Feshbach 1986). These programs often use role playing to help students learn about perspective-taking and to practice resolving interpersonal conflicts, and have proven effective in increasing children's caring behaviors, self-conceptions, and social understanding (Eisenberg 1992: 116–17). Closely related to empathy-training programs but somewhat broader are emotional literacy courses. While people often assume that children develop their emotions naturally, researchers have come to recognize that our emotions need to be cultivated and taught just like our other basic capabilities (Goleman 1995). If children are not encouraged to identify, express, and regulate their different emotions and not provided a vocabulary to discuss them—as happens more often to boys than girls—they 'may become largely unconscious of their emotional states, both in themselves and others' (Brody and Hall 1993: 456; see also Nussbaum 2001: 150). Lacking an awareness of their own emotions and those of others, children may have difficulty sympathizing with others and responding to them in sensitive ways. Emotional education should therefore be added to the elementary school curriculum in order to foster more caring dispositions in children. As with empathy training programs, emotional literacy programs have proven effective in promoting emotional understanding and pro-social and caring behaviors, while also increasing academic achievement scores and decreasing the risk of antisocial and aggressive behavior (Goleman 1995: 261–87, 305–9; Kusche and Greenberg 2001: 152–6). Many of these programs can be easily integrated into already existing courses in writing, social studies, science, and other traditional disciplines, and hence would not involve establishing new classes.

The educational system can also play a crucial role in broadening children's sense of sympathy and compassion for individuals who are different from them. Even children who receive attentive care from their parents may grow up to have a relatively constricted view of caring unless conscious efforts are made to expand their moral horizons. One reason many Americans currently oppose certain welfare programs, for example, is because they hold negative stereotypes of racial minorities whom they regard as the primary beneficiaries of these programs (Gilens 1999). There are numerous ways that schools might attempt to address the racial attitudes of students, including racial sensitivity programs, but one important step would be to teach diverse perspectives in history and literature classes with the goal of cultivating a sense

231

of sympathy and unity among students. Jorge Valadez argues in this regard that multicultural education should include both informative and affective dimensions (Valadez 2001: 94–6). The informative dimensions would include learning about the history of different groups so that individuals outside any particular group can better understand the prominent perspectives and concerns of individuals within the group. The affective dimension would include reading important works of literature and viewing works of art by individuals from diverse backgrounds. Courses in American literature might expose students to the experiences and perspectives of Anglo-Americans, African-Americans, Mexican-Americans, Asian-Americans, and others, and encourage students to identify with the problems, hopes, and dreams of the main characters in these books. As distinct from many of the usual justifications for multicultural education, the goal here would be to expand students' sympathy and compassion for individuals who are not like them rather than to provide recognition to different groups in society. If trade-offs must be made regarding what is to be taught, it is therefore probably better to provide students with an in-depth introduction to the experiences and perspectives of one or two groups rather than barraging them with a superficial knowledge of many cultures.

History and social studies courses might further contribute to the development of more sympathetic and caring students in other ways. These courses might, for example, give more emphasis to personal acts of caring and altruism in world affairs (Oliner 1979, 1983, 1985–6). When government and history classes focus solely on institutional processes and world historical events, students are likely to see the driving forces of human affairs as war, self-interest, and material gain and to overlook the important role played by individual acts of benevolence and care in shaping world affairs. The Holocaust, for example, is not just the story of Nazis killing Jews, but also of Jewish courage in the face of adversity and individuals helping Jews to escape from Nazis. Examples of courage and care are important in history for teaching students about the power of individual sympathy and compassion to bring about change.

A final possible curriculum reform at the high school level might be the addition of a service learning course. All students might be required to take at least one course during their high school careers that engages them directly in some form of caring work. They could be transported for several hours each week to perform volunteer work at a community organization, or taken to a nearby elementary school to tutor young

232

students in reading and math. Alternatively, schools could design service learning programs on their own campuses that engage students in helping others or organizing events in the community. Coordinating service learning courses is usually difficult, and if students cannot be engaged in meaningful community projects, then it is probably best that schools not initiate these programs at all. The last thing one wants to do is to send a message to students that community work is frivolous and inconsequential. However, when it is possible to institute meaningful service learning programs, it seems important to try to do so. These programs can provide students with important practice in caring for others and tend to promote pro-social behavior later in life (Eisenberg and Fabes 1998: 720–21).

If the American education system is to succeed at achieving the most basic aim of caring—namely, developing children's basic capabilities and preparing them for life in society—it will require much more wide-ranging reforms than anything discussed here. At present, far too many students never learn to read, write, perform basic math, express themselves, or reason clearly in American schools. Any number of educational reform proposals might be appropriate to address these shortcomings. The discussion here has focused more narrowly on the question of how the American education system might be made more supportive of caring values and attitudes. In this regard, no major overhaul of educational practices or curriculum seems necessary. A change of emphasis in pedagogy, the addition of social emotional learning programs, a more effective multicultural education, and a more concerted effort to integrate caring ideals into existing courses would likely help students to develop more caring dispositions. These reforms admittedly do nothing to teach students life skills such as parenting, cooking, budgeting, and so forth, but having taken some of these classes in high school, I must admit to being skeptical about their value. Unless students are already living on their own or are engaged in parenting, they are unlikely to view these courses as relevant or interesting. Rather than requiring students to take these courses before they have a direct need for them, it might be better if the government offered parenting and other life skill classes (perhaps at local high schools) as free adult education classes for new parents or anyone else interested in taking them. In high school, it is probably more important simply to try to encourage students to think beyond themselves and to encourage them to develop more caring attitudes than to provide them with parenting or home skills that they may not yet be ready to use.

## 5.5. Caring and the Media

The media are another cultural institution with a potentially powerful influence on people's attitudes and behaviors. The media include television, movies, radio, music, newspapers, video games, the Internet, and other entertainment and information sources. Since it would be far too great a task to consider all the different media here, I will focus on the effects of television on people's attitudes about caring.[22]

Most research on television has focused on its negative effects, but television programming can also contribute to caring and pro-social behaviors (Eisenberg 1992: 129–30; Silk 1998; Urslaner 1998). Many television programs depict acts of caring and kindness and portray nurturing and supportive relationships in a positive and attractive light. News stories and documentaries often draw attention to the needs of individuals and communities and frequently elicit caring responses from the public. In these respects, television can, and in many cases does, encourage individuals to attend to and take responsibility for the needs of others.

In various other ways, however, television viewing appears to undermine caring attitudes and behaviors. A number of longitudinal studies have found that childhood exposure to television violence correlates with, or may even cause, more aggressive behaviors in young adults (Huesmann and Miller 1994; Huesmann, Moise, and Podolski 1997; Huesmann et al. 2003). Other studies have demonstrated that individuals who have been exposed to violent programming are slower to react to real world violence and less sympathetic to the victims of violence (Donnerstein, Linz, and Penrod 1987; Drabman and Thomas 1975; Grossman and Degaetano 1999; Linz, Donnerstein, and Penrod 1988). Researchers have also argued that heavy television viewing can cultivate a sense of anxiety and fear in individuals that may incline them to be less sympathetic and more punitive toward others (Gerbner 1992, 1995; Heath and Gilbert 1996; Morgan and Shanahan 1997; Potter 2003: 146–8; Signorielli 1990). Critics have challenged this research by pointing out flaws in the methodologies and noting that the negative effects of television violence are only modest (Fowles 1999; Freedman 2002; Uslaner 1998). Nonetheless, a substantial number of studies have found that television violence at least correlates with higher levels of aggression and can lead to insensitivity and fear in at

---

[22] For a synopsis of recent research on the effects of television on child development, see Huston and Wright 1998.

least some individuals, and even modest increases in people's tendencies toward aggressiveness, desensitization, and fear can have dramatic consequences when multiplied over the whole of society (Bushman and Anderson 2001, 482; Potter 2003: 27–9, 31–51).

Television may also contribute to harmful stereotypes that incline individuals to be less sympathetic to others. Media news stories tend to overrepresent African-Americans in stories about poverty and welfare, which appears to contribute to many Americans' opposition to welfare programs (Gilens 1999; Iyengar 1991). Television also appears to perpetuate gender stereotypes and sexualized images of women (Brody 1999: 238–40; Herrett-Skjellum and Allen 1996; Huston and Wright 1998: 1035–7; Shields 1997). Men are generally depicted in higher status roles and as more powerful than women in television programs, and women are often portrayed as subordinate and sex objects. There is, in turn, a strong correlation between television watching and sexist attitudes: 'very sexist persons are twice as likely also to be heavy viewers of television' (Herrett-Skjellum and Allen 1996: 178). Some experimental studies have further found that men who are exposed to sexually explicit materials are more likely to endorse violence against women, express less compassion for female rape victims, and report a greater willingness to force women into sexual acts (Check and Guloien 1989; Malamuth and Check 1981; Pally 1994; Zillmann and Bryant 1982). Once again, however, this research remains controversial.[23]

Television may also take time away from personal and communal forms of caring. Roughly half of all Americans report watching television while eating dinner, and nearly one-third watch television during breakfast and lunch. Eighty-one percent of Americans say they watch television most evenings, while only fifty-six percent report talking with family members (Putnam 2000: 227–8). Husbands and wives spend on average three to four times more time watching television than they spend talking to one other (Putnam 2000: 224). In *Bowling Alone*, Robert Putnam draws upon this data to argue that heavy television viewing is one of the major causes of the decline of civic engagement in the United States over the last fifty years (Putnam 2000: 216–46). The more time people spend watching television, the less time they have to attend public meetings, serve in local

[23] A number of studies have found that while exposure to violent imagery increases aggression toward women, nonviolent sexual material appears to generate no aggressive effects (Donnerstein, Linz, and Penrod 1988; Pally 1994: 42–7). It therefore seems questionable that sexually explicit material causes violence against women, but it probably does reinforce sexual stereotypes that may make men less sympathetic to women's concerns.

organizations, and join clubs.[24] Caring for others involves a narrower and slightly different set of activities than civic engagement, but there are at least some good intuitive reasons for thinking that television might have a similarly negative impact on the quantity and quality of caring that individuals give to one another. If parents are spending a great deal of time watching television rather than personally engaging with their children, and children are spending a great deal of time watching television alone rather than engaging with their parents or friends, then it goes to reason that television might take time away from caring practices.

Television can be criticized on other grounds, but the focus here is on its effects on people's proclivity to care for others. While the evidence supporting the view that television makes people less sympathetic and caring is controversial, there does seem to be some reason for concern. Many television programs do appear to encourage violence and decrease sympathy and compassion in at least some number of people. A caring society, then, would seemingly want to do something at least to mitigate the potentially harmful effects that television may have on individuals' dispositions to care.

Virginia Held has outlined one plan for developing a more caring media (Held 1988; 1993: 91–111). Held argues that many of the negative effects of the media can be traced back to its commercialized nature. 'The culture of the marketplace has often reinforced sexual and racial stereotypes, presenting women's bodies as objects to be bought and sold and used and discarded; it has made violence and domination sexually charged and appealing, and in its portrayals of social realities has often distorted and obscured them in damaging ways' (1993: 97). Since violence and sex sell, market-driven media sources gravitate toward programs with this content. Her solution is 'a massive effort, comparable to that which brought about our system of public education, to publicly fund the production of noncommercial culture, including mass culture' (Held 1993: 107–8; see also Held 1988 and most recently Held 2006: 122). Private broadcasters and publishers would continue to exist in this plan, but they would be supplemented by a broad range of publicly funded, noncommercial alternatives including public television stations, public production companies, public newspapers, and so on. Divorced from commercial pressures, Held suggests that public production companies would create more diverse and higher quality programs, and public television and radio stations

[24] Uslaner among others has challenged Putnam's thesis on the grounds that there is no clear empirical evidence showing that television reduces civic participation (1998, 2002).

would air more diverse and enriching programs. The government would raise money for public media sources by taxing commercial broadcasters and advertisers. To protect against government interference, Held further suggests that independent media boards could be established to manage public media apart from direct governmental oversight (1988: 172).

Held's proposal has some obvious merits, but is probably not the best solution for addressing the problems outlined above. On the one hand, even if writers, producers, actors, and others were freed from market pressures, there is no guarantee that they would produce more caring programming. They might simply produce more stylized sex and violence, as many independent filmmakers currently do. On the other hand, Held's solution is extremely costly given the apparently limited effects that the media—or at least television—has on people's dispositions. Public funding for television, movies, newspapers, and other media sources would cost billions of dollars each year, and the more successful public broadcasters were in attracting large audiences for their programs, the less tax revenue would be available from private broadcast companies to fund these programs. Held's core point about more public funding for the media is nonetheless a good one. Studies suggest that the media can be used to promote sympathy, caring, cooperation, and other pro-social attitudes and behaviors (Eisenberg 1992: 129–30). Yet more limited measures are probably called for. Rather than bringing a large part of the media under public ownership and control, the government might offer more public funding for the development of programs that model caring behaviors and foster sympathy and compassion for others. Direct grants would ensure that programs were developed for the specific purpose of promoting caring values and would be less costly than creating new production companies and stations. Since the overall effect of this reform would likely be small, however, other measures would also be necessary.

A second way the government might try to mitigate the negative effects of television would be to exercise more direct regulation over television broadcasting. In England, Australia, and many other countries, regulations exist that forbid broadcasters from showing violent programs during times when children are most likely to be watching television. In the United States, such safe viewing laws may not be constitutional, but if clear guidelines were developed for censoring only those forms of television violence that research has shown to be most harmful to viewers—actions that glamorize, sanitize, and trivialize violence—then they might pass constitutional review (Potter 2003: 85–102, 140–52). W. James Potter among others is nonetheless skeptical about the effectiveness of safe viewing laws, since many children are still watching programs at nine or ten o'clock at night and television violence affects not only children but also adolescents and adults (Potter 2003: 67–84, 169). Even so, banishing violent programs to the late hours would at least decrease the amount of harmful violence that children, adolescents, and adults view on television and reduce the overall number of violent programs that are produced.

A third measure for mitigating the harmful effects of television and other media on people would be for the government to mandate and fund media literacy courses for all students in public schools. Several organizations have developed extensive media literacy programs, and countries such as England, Australia, and Canada already teach media literacy in their schools (Huston and Wright 1998: 1042; Potter 2003: 189–94). It is frankly astonishing that in a media saturated society such as the United States, media studies courses are not already mandated in all public schools. The basic goal of most media literacy courses is to help students to gain a critical awareness of television programming and to distinguish reality from fantasy. Courses might begin early by asking young students to engage in activities such as counting the number of violent acts in a program and then discussing nonviolent ways in which characters might have resolved their problems. Older students might study gender and racial stereotypes in the media, and compare actual crime rates and violence in their communities with the number of news stories devoted to these topics. Students might also learn about the commercial nature of the media and explore the effects of media violence on people. If successful, these courses could combat many of television's undesirable effects by making people more critical of the programs they view. Individuals who came to recognize television violence as gratuitous and as disproportionate to the violence in society, for example, would likely be less aggressive, suspicious, and punitive toward others in society.

The final practical reform actually has little to do directly with television itself, and hence is often overlooked by media scholars. If heavy television viewing contributes even in small ways to aggression, fear, racism, or sexism, or takes time away from caring activities, then the best response would seem to be to encourage people to watch less television. Short of highly authoritarian measures, little can be done to change the habits of people who have already become habituated to heavy television viewing. Steps can be taken, however, to encourage children to watch less television, and one means for doing so would be to provide support for childcare centers and after school programs. Publicly subsidized childcare centers and after school programs would both decrease the amount of time children spend watching television (assuming that television viewing was discouraged in these programs), and increase the likelihood that they would become interested in other activities such as reading or sports that would keep them from watching so much television. Reducing the amount of time young children and adolescents spend watching television by even one hour each day could have significant long-term effects on their levels of aggression, fear, racism, and sexism, and would generally habituate them to watch less television over the course of their lives.

These reforms are relatively minor and obviously would not counteract all the negative effects associated with television viewing, but they would at least mitigate them. In a culture that values free expression and individual choice, it seems that little more can be done in a cost-effective manner. Moreover, it is important to keep in perspective that television viewing appears to have relatively minor effects on people's attitudes and behaviors, and thus does not seem to warrant drastic measures. If the other reforms discussed in this chapter were implemented (subsidized parental leaves, quality childcare centers, etc.), it seems likely that in the long run people would in any case become more sympathetic and caring and would be less affected by whatever violent, sexist, or racially stereotypical programming they might see. In the final analysis, these other reforms are probably the most important measures for addressing the negative effects of television. If we change the attitudes of people so that they are more positively disposed toward caring for others, they will be less likely to be negatively effected by violent and prejudicial programming, and eventually television programming might even change to reflect the kinder and gentler views of most people.

## 5.6. Conclusion

The cultural institutions that currently exist in the United States virtually ensure that many individuals grow up with a limited sense of sympathy and compassion for others and little motivation to care for others beyond their immediate family and friends. Lack of support for parenting leaves and early childhood education means that many children never develop the basic trust and sympathy necessary for broadly caring attitudes and behaviors. The gendered division of care work subtly encourages many boys and men to distance themselves from caring activities and social policies. The absence of social emotional learning courses and empathy training in many schools leaves many children's capability for sympathy and compassion underdeveloped. The government's limited efforts to regulate television viewing further reinforces a culture of violence and mistrust.

The reforms outlined in this chapter all provide practical measures for increasing individuals' dispositions to care. None of these reforms is especially radical or intrusive, but all would increase the likelihood that more individuals would develop the sorts of sympathetic and compassionate dispositions that would make them more inclined to support caring institutions and policies. Many of these reforms would also have positive social consequences quite apart from fostering more caring individuals. Emotional learning courses, for example, not only foster more sympathetic and compassionate individuals but also tend to increase academic performance, self-control, cooperation, and other socially beneficial traits. Adequate care for young children has similarly positive effects. People thus might agree to support these measures for self-interested reasons. Their long-term effect would nonetheless likely be an increase in the number of people who recognize caring as a public good and feel motivated to support and comply with caring institutions and policies. In this way, these reforms would help to nudge individuals toward developing the emotions and disposition that ultimately underlie a caring theory of justice.

# Conclusion

In this book, I have developed care ethics into a theory of justice and situated it in relation to other contemporary justice theories. Beginning with a general definition of caring practices and an account of our obligation to care for others, I have outlined the basic institutions and policies of a caring society in the domains of domestic politics, economics, international relations, and culture. I have also engaged care ethics in current debates about multiculturalism and cultural relativism. While this book has covered a lot of ground, I am nonetheless struck here at the end by how much more work still remains to be done in developing a moral and political theory of caring. I have undoubtedly overlooked some policies that might be useful in supporting caring practices at home or abroad, and have admittedly addressed several important topics (such as care theory and education and care theory and the media) in only a cursory way. Moreover, since the focus of this book has been on general institutions and policies, many particular issues, such as care theory's approach to crime and punishment, the environment, and immigration, also remain to be further explored. My goal in this book has been not so much to provide a discussion of all the institutions and policies that flow from care theory as to outline a general framework for thinking about why we should and how we might care for others through our political and social institutions.

Many countries already support many of the policies discussed in this book. Over the past fifty years, many countries have passed parental leave policies, established public childcare centers, and implemented universal health programs. Political theory has, however, generally lagged behind political practice in recognizing and justifying these policies. In Marxian terms, we might say that the material conditions of society have outstripped our social and political vision. Demographic, economic, and other changes in society have created a need for public policies that support and accommodate caring policies, but many political theorists continue to treat society as essentially unchanged. When one turns to the major works of political theory written over the last half century—say, Rawls's *A Theory of Justice*—one finds no mention of many caring policies and only oblique references to many others. Moreover, the major schools of contemporary political thought—including liberalism, communitarianism, and to a lesser extent natural law theory—are not especially well suited for recognizing and justifying many caring policies. While politicians have thus found themselves in recent years responding to the very real needs of individuals for more caring policies, political theorists have generally ignored these developments or failed to recognize them as representing anything new, except perhaps for libertarian theorists who have generally heaped scorn upon them. Care theory recasts and justifies these political developments as constituting the emergence of a new understanding of the nature and purpose of government. It specifically offers a new theory of justice that can guide and justify the development of a new form of welfare state organized around the fundamental goal of supporting and accommodating caring practices.

While some countries already provide support for caring practices, other countries, such as the United States, currently provide very little support for these practices. In these countries, a political theory of caring represents a fairly radical and new vision of what government can and should do. Care theory does not, however, call for anything like a revolutionary struggle to implement a new caring regime. Rather, it lends itself nicely to a gradualist or piecemeal approach to reform. If governments were to pass even a few caring policies, the long-term effect would likely be a citizen body more supportive of additional caring policies. By establishing universal health care or elder care policies, for example, governments would generate more generalized trust and caring dispositions among people that would make people more likely to support future caring programs (Rothstein and Uslaner 2005). By guaranteeing all people subsidized parental leaves and quality childcare, governments would likewise do more than just contribute to the immediate well-being of parents and children; they would also plant the seeds of a more caring citizenry.

Most of the arguments for a caring political theory in this book have been either of a moral or prudential nature. Above all, I have argued that we all have a duty to care for others rooted in our nature as dependent creatures. Our dependency on others for care implicitly commits us to a morality of caring for others in need. Capable individuals violate their own implicit morality (and for most people, commonsense moral intuitions) when they refuse to care for other needy individuals. I have also highlighted some of the self-interested reasons for supporting a caring government. Good care for children generally translates into more well adjusted, capable, and productive adults, and less aggression, violence, and unemployment throughout society. Good health care for all people means a healthier and more productive populace, lower risks of infectious diseases, and lower overall medical costs. Since many of us will further find ourselves at some point sick, disabled, or otherwise in need of care, and most of us have parents, grandparents, children, siblings, friends, or others who will require care, we also all have an interest in establishing general caring policies. The best way to ensure that we and our loved ones will receive adequate care when necessary is by establishing social policies that guarantee adequate care to all individuals. We are all likely to benefit both directly and indirectly from general caring policies.

There is also one other important reason for caring for others that has not received much attention in my argument: caring is a good in itself. Many parents consider the care they provide for their children to be the most fulfilling and meaningful activity of their lives. Individuals who devote themselves to the care of a sick or disabled spouse, friend, child, or stranger sometimes arrive at a new, almost spiritual understanding of themselves and their connection to others. Even just performing a simple act of caring for another can stimulate a temporary sense of contentment and joy.

The good we feel in caring for others can be related back to our own dependent existence. The Dalai Lama writes in this regard:

We humans are social beings. We come into the world as the result of others' actions. We survive here in dependence on others. Whether we like it or not, there is hardly a moment of our lives when we do not benefit from others' activities. For this reason, it is hardly surprising that most of our happiness arises in the context of our relationships with others. Nor is it so remarkable that our greatest joy should come when we are motivated by concern for others. (1999: 62)

When we care for others, we repay our most basic moral debt to others. We care for others as others have cared for us. In doing so, we experience humanity at its most vulnerable and discover in ourselves the generative power to sustain and reproduce human life. It is not only the Dalai Lama who has seen in caring the key to a happy life, but also other writers such as Martin Buber (1970) and Emmanuel Levinas

243

(1969) who have argued that caring for others provides a bridge to the divine.[1]

Caring for others on a political level is different from personally caring for a child or friend, but there is no reason why political caring should affect us differently from personal caring. The willful neglect or ignorance of the needs of distant others does not make them go away, but means only that we have shut ourselves off from others and (by extension) from the full recognition of our own humanity. When we turn our backs on others in need, we turn our backs in part on ourselves. We refuse to recognize in the needs of others the dependency that exists within all of us. It is only by expanding our caring beyond our circle of family and friends and extending it to all others in need that we ultimately come to recognize our universal human self and experience our interdependency with all other human beings. We then come to know ourselves as dependent creatures who share with all other human beings a common need for the care of other human beings, and discover the morality that lies at the heart of human existence: caring.

---

[1] For a discussion of the relationship between care ethics and Buber, see Noddings (1984: 17, 32, 73–4, *passim*). For a discussion of the relationship between care ethics and Levinas, see Groenhout (2004: 79–103).

# Bibliography

Administration for Children and Families (2001). 'IN FOCUS: Understanding the Effects of Maltreatment on Early Brain Development'. Washington, DC: US Department of Health and Human Services. Available at http://nccanch.acf.hhs. gov/pubs/focus/earlybrain.cfm

Agarwal, Archana (2005). 'Violence against Women: The Problems Confronting International Human Rights Law, Comprehending the Injuries and Conceptualizing the Remedies'. Paper presented at the Western Political Science Association Annual Meeting. Oakland, CA.

Ainsworth, Mary, Mary Blehar, Everett Waters, and Sally Wall (1978). *Patterns of Attachment: A Psychological Study of the Strange Situation.* Hillsdale, NJ: Erlbaum.

Albelda, Randy (2004). 'An Immodest Proposal', *Feminist Economics*, 10(2): 251–8.

—— Nancy Folbre, and the Center for Popular Economics (1996). *The War on the Poor: A Defense Manual.* New York: New Press.

Alstott, Anne (2004). *No Exit: What Parents Owe Their Children and What Society Owes Parents.* Oxford: Oxford University Press.

An-Na'im, Abdullahi Ahmed (1990). *Toward and Islamic Reformation: Civil Liberties, Human Rights, and International Law.* Syracuse, NY: Syracuse University Press.

Aristotle (1995). *The Politics*, trans. Ernest Barker. Oxford: Oxford University Press.

Baier, Annette (1985). *Pictures of the Mind: Essays on Mind and Morals.* Minneapolis, MN: University of Minnesota Press.

—— (1994). *Moral Prejudices: Essays on Ethics.* Cambridge, MA: Harvard University Press.

—— (1997). *The Commons of the Mind.* Chicago, IL: Open Court.

Bailyn, Lotte (1993). *Breaking the Mold.* New York: Free Press.

Baker, Dean and Mark Weisbrot (2001). *Social Security: The Phony Crisis.* Chicago, IL: University of Chicago Press.

Barrett, Christopher and Daniel Maxwell (2005). *Food Aid After Fifty Years: Recasting Its Role.* New York: Routledge.

Barry, Brian (1995). *Justice as Impartiality.* Oxford: Oxford University Press.

—— (2001). *Culture and Equality: An Egalitarian Critique of Multiculturalism.* Cambridge, MA: Harvard University Press.

—— (2005). *Why Social Justice Matters.* Cambridge: Polity Press.

Bar-Tal, Daniel (1976). *Prosocial Behavior: Theory and Research.* New York: John Wiley and Sons.

Beitz, Charles (1979). *Political Theory and International Relations.* Princeton, NJ: Princeton University Press.

Bell, Daniel (2000). *East Meets West: Human Rights and Democracy in East Asia.* Princeton, NJ: Princeton University Press.

—— and Joseph Carens. (2004). 'The Ethical Dilemmas of International Human Rights and Humanitarian NGOs: Reflections on a Dialogue between Practitioners and Theorists', *Human Rights Quarterly*, 26: 300–29.

Beneria, Lourdes (2003). *Gender, Development, and Globalization.* New York: Routledge.

Benhabib, Seyla (2002). *The Claims of Culture: Equality and Diversity in the Global Era.* Princeton, NJ: Princeton University Press.

Berkowitz, Leonard (1993). *Aggression: Its Causes, Consequences, and Control.* Philadelphia, PA: Temple University Press.

Beyleveld, Deryck (1991). *The Dialectical Necessity of Morality: An Analysis and Defense of Alan Gewirth's Argument to the Principle of Generic Consistency.* Chicago, IL: University of Chicago Press.

Bhavnagri, Navaz Peshotan and Janet Gonzalez-Mena (1997). 'The Cultural Context of Infant Caregiving', *Childhood Education*, 74 (Fall): 2–8.

Birdsall, Nancy, Dani Rodrik, and Arvind Subramanian (2005). *Foreign Affairs*, 84(4) (July/August): 136–52.

Blankenhorn, David (1995). *Fatherless America.* New York: Basic Books.

Blau, David (2001). *The Child Care Problem: An Economic Analysis.* New York: Russell Sage Foundation.

Block, Fred (2001). 'Introduction', in Karl Polanyied (ed.), *The Great Transformation: The Political and Economic Origins of Our Time.* Boston, MA: Beacon Press.

Blum, Lawrence (1994). *Moral Perception and Particularity.* Cambridge: Cambridge University Press.

Blustein, Jeffrey (1991). *Care and Commitment: Taking the Personal Point of View.* Oxford: Oxford University Press.

Bond, E. J (1980). 'Gewirth on Reason and Morality', *Metaphilosophy*, 11(1): 36–53.

Bowden, Peta (1997). *Caring: Gender-Sensitive Ethics.* London: Routledge.

Bowlby, John (1969). *Attachment and Loss. Volume I: Attachment.* London: Hogarth Press and the Institute of Psychoanalysis.

—— (1973). *Attachment and Loss. Volume II: Separation: Anxiety and Anger.* New York: Basic Books.

—— (1980). *Attachment and Loss. Volume III: Loss: Sadness and Depression.* New York: Basic Books.

—— (1988). *A Secure Base: Parent-Child Attachment and Healthy Human Development.* New York: Basic Books.

Braybrooke, David (1987). *Meeting Needs*. Princeton, NJ: Princeton University Press.

Brody, Leslie (1999). *Gender, Emotion, and the Family*. Cambridge, MA: Harvard University Press.

—— and Judith Hall (1993). 'Gender and Emotion', in Michael Lewis and Jeannette Haviland (eds), *Handbook of Emotions*. New York: Guildford Press.

Brown, Chris (2002). *Sovereignty, Rights and Justice: International Political Theory Today*. Cambridge: Polity.

Brown, J. Larry and Ernesto Pollitt (1996).'Malnutrition, Poverty and Intellectual Development', *Scientific American*, (February): 38–43.

Bubeck, Diemut (1995). *Care, Gender, and Justice*. Oxford: Clarendon Press.

Buber, Martin (1970). *I and Thou*. Trans. Walter Kaufmann. New York: Simon and Schuster.

Buchanan, Allen (2003*a*). *Justice, Legitimacy, and Self-Determination: Moral Foundations for International Law*. Oxford: Oxford University Press.

—— (2003*b*). 'Reforming the International Law of Humanitarian Intervention', in J. L. Holzgrege and Robert Keohane (eds), *Humanitarian Intervention: Ethical, Legal, and Political Dilemmas*. Cambridge: Cambridge University Press, pp. 130–73.

Bushman, Brad and Craig Anderson (2001). 'Media Violence and the American Public: Scientific Facts versus Media Misinformation', *American Psychologist*, 56(6/7) (June/July): 477–89.

Campbell, F. A., C. T. Ramey, E. P. Pungello, J. Sparling, and S. Miller-Johnson (2002). 'Early Childhood Education: Young Adult Outcomes from the Abecedarian Project', *Applied Developmental Science*, 6: 42–57.

Cancian, Francesca and Stacey Oliker (2000). *Caring and Gender*. Walnut Creek, CA: Alta Mira Press.

Card, Claudia (1990). 'Caring and Evil', *Hypatia* 5 (Spring): 101–08.

Card, David and Alan Krueger (1995). *Myth and Measurement: The New Economics for the Minimum Wage*. Princeton, NJ: Princeton University Press.

—— —— (1999). 'A Reanalysis of the Effect of the New Jersey Minimum Wage Increase on the Fast-Food Industry with Representative Payroll Data', Working Paper No. 393. Princeton University. Available at http://ideas.repec.org/p/fth/prinin/393.html

Carlson, Bonnie (1984). 'The Father's Contribution to Child Care: Effects on Children's Perception of Parental Role', *American Journal of Orthopsychology*, 54: 123–36.

Check, J. V. P. and T. H. Guloien (1989). 'Reported Proclivity for Coercive Sex following Repeated Exposure to Sexually Violent Pornography, Nonviolent Pornography, and Erotica', in D. Zillmann and J. Bryant (eds), *Pornography: Research Advances and Policy Considerations*. Hillsdale, NJ: Lawrence Erlbaum Associates, pp. 159–84.

Chesterman, Simon (2001). *Just War or Just Peace? Humanitarian Intervention and International Law*. Oxford: Oxford University Press.

Chodorow, Nancy (1978). *The Reproduction of Mothering: Psychoanalysis and the Sociology of Gender*. Berkeley, CA: University of California Press.

—— (1994). *Feminities, Masculinities, Sexualities: Freud and Beyond*. Kentucky: University Press of Kentucky.

—— (1999). *The Reproduction of Mothering: Psychoanalysis and the Sociology of Gender*, 2nd edn, Berkeley, CA: University of California Press.

Christopher, Paul (2004). *The Ethics of War and Peace: An Introduction to Legal and Moral Issues*, 3rd edn, Upper Saddle River, NJ: Pearson.

Clement, Grace (1996). *Care, Autonomy, and Justice*. Boulder, CO: Westview Press.

Code, Lorraine (1987*a*). *Epistemic Responsibility*. Hanover, New Hampshire: University Press of New England.

—— (1987*b*). 'Second Persons', in Marsha Hanen and Kai Nielsen (eds), *Science, Morality and Feminist Theory. Supplementary Volume of the Canadian Journal of Philosophy*. Calgary, Canada: University of Calgary Press, pp. 357–82.

Cohen, Jean and Andrew Arato (1992). *Civil Society and Political Theory*. Cambridge, MA: MIT Press.

Cohen, Jonathan (ed.) (2001). *Caring Classrooms/Intelligent Schools: The Social Emotional Education of Young Children*. New York: Teachers College Press.

Cohen, Joshua (2004). 'Minimalism About Human Rights: The Most We Can Hope For?', *The Journal of Political Philosophy*, 12(2): 190–213.

Collins, Patricia Hill (2000). *Black Feminist Thought: Knowledge, Consciousness, and the Politics of Empowerment*, 2nd edn, New York: Routledge.

Crittenden, Paul (1990). *Learning to be Moral: Philosophical Thoughts about Moral Development*. New Jersey: Humanities Press International.

Cubed, M. (2002). 'The National Economic Impacts of the Child Care Sector'. Available at http://www.nccanet.org/NCCA%20Impact%20Study.pdf

Dalai Lama (1999). *Ethics for the New Millennium*. New York: Riverhead Books.

Dalla Costa, Mariarosa and Selma James (1975). *The Power of Women and the Subversion of the Community*. Bristol, UK: Falling Wall Press.

Damasio, Antonio (1994). *Descartes' Error: Emotion, Reason, and the Human Brain*. New York: HarperCollins.

Damon, William (1988). *The Moral Child: Nurturing Children's Natural Moral Growth*. New York: Free Press.

Darwall, Stephen (2002). *Welfare and Rational Care*. Princeton, NJ: Princeton University Press.

Dasho, Stefan, Catherine Lewis, and Marilyn Watson (2001). 'Fostering Emotional Intelligence in the Classroom and School: Strategies from the Child Development Project', in Jonathan Cohen (ed.), *Caring Classrooms/Intelligent Schools: The Social Emotional Education of Young Children*. New York: Teachers College Press, pp. 87–107.

De Waal, Alexander (1997). *Famine Crimes: Politics and the Disaster Relief Industry in Africa*. Bloomington, IN: Indiana University Press.

Dietz, Mary (1985). 'The Problem with Maternal Thinking'. *Political Theory*, 13(1) (February): 19–37.

Diller, Ann (1996). 'The Ethics of Care and Education: A New Paradigm, Its Critics, and Its Educational Significance', in Ann Diller, Barbara Houston, Kathryn Pauly Morgan, and Maryann Ayim (eds), *The Gender Question in Education: Theory, Pedagogy, and Politics*. Boulder, CO: Westview, pp. 89–104.

Donath, Susan (2000). 'The Other Economy: A Suggestion for a Distinctively Feminist Economics', *Feminist Economics* 6(1): 115–23.

Donnelly, Jack (1989). *Universal Human Rights in Theory and Practice*. Ithaca: Cornell University Press.

—— (2003). *Universal Human Rights in Theory and Practice*, 2nd edn, Ithaca, NY: Cornell University Press.

Donnerstein, Edward, Daniel Linz, and Steven Penrod (1987). *The Question of Pornography: Research Findings and Policy Implications*. New York: Free Press.

Donovan, Josephine (1996). 'Attention to Suffering: Sympathy as a Basis for the Ethical Treatment of Animals', in Josephine Donovan and Carol Adams (eds), *Beyond Animal Rights: A Feminist Caring Ethic for the Treatment of Animals*. New York: Continuum.

Doyle, Michael (2006). 'One World, Many Peoples: International Justice in John Rawls's *The Law of Peoples*'. *Perspectives on Politics*, 4(1) (March): 109–20.

Drabman, R. S. and M. H. Thomas (1975). 'Does TV Violence Breed Indifference?', *Journal of Communication*, 25: 86–89.

Duindam, Vincent and Ed Spruijt (2002). 'The Reproduction of Fathering', *Feminism and Psychology*, 12: 28–32.

Easterly, William (2001). *The Elusive Quest for Growth: Economists' Adventures and Misadventures in the Tropics*. Cambridge, MA: MIT Press.

—— (2006). *The White Man's Burden: Why the West's Efforts to Aid the Rest Have Done So Much Ill and So Little Good*. New York: Penguin.

Eisenberg, Nancy (1992). *The Caring Child*. Cambridge, MA: Harvard University Press.

—— and Richard Fabes (1998). 'Prosocial Development', in William Damon and Nancy Eisenberg (eds), *Handbook of Child Psychology. Volume Three: Social, Emotional, and Personality Development*. New York: John Wiley and Sons, pp. 701–78.

El-Affendi, Abdelwahab (2001). 'Islam and Human Rights: The Lessons from Sudan', *Muslim World*, 91(3/4): 481–506

Elicker, J., M. Englund, and L. A. Sroufe (1992). 'Predicting Peer Competence and Peer Relationships in Childhood from Early Parent-Child Relationships', in R. D. Parke and G. W. Ladd (eds), *Family-peer Relationships: Modes of Linkage*. Hillsdale, NJ: Erlbaum, pp. 77–106.

England, Paula, Michelle Budig, and Nancy Folbre (2002). 'Wages of Virtue: The Relative Pay of Care Work', *Social Problems*, 49(4): 455–73.

Engster, Daniel (2001). 'Mary Wollstonecraft's Nurturing Liberalism: Between an Ethic of Justice and Care', *American Political Science Review*, 95(3) (September): 577–88.

—— (2004). 'Care Ethics and Natural Law Theory: Toward an Institutional Political Theory of Caring', *The Journal of Politics*, 66(1) (February): 113–35.

—— (2007). 'Care Ethics and Animal Welfare', *Journal of Social Philosophy*, 37(4): 521–36.

Etzioni, Amitai (1993). *The Spirit of Community: The Reinvention of American Society.* New York: Simon and Schuster.

Falk, Richard (1999). *Predatory Globalization: A Critique.* Polity Press.

Feinberg, Joel (1970a). *Doing and Deserving: Essays in the Theory of Responsibility.* Princeton, NJ: Princeton University Press.

—— (1970b). 'The Nature and Value of Rights', *The Journal of Value Inquiry*, 4(4) (Winter): 243–60.

Feshbach, N. D (1982). 'Sex Differences in Empathy and Social Behavior in Children', in Nancy Eisenberg (ed.), *The Development of Prosocial Behavior.* New York: Academic Press.

Feshbach, S. and N. D. Feshbach (1986). 'Aggression and Altruism: A Personality Perspective', in C. Zahn-Waxler, E. M. Cummings, and R. Iannotti (eds), *Altruism and Aggression: Biological and Social Origins.* Cambridge: Cambridge University Press, pp. 189–217.

Fineman, Martha (1995). *The Neutered Mother, the Sexual Family and Other Twentieth Century Tragedies.* New York: Routledge.

—— (2004). *The Autonomy Myth: A Theory of Dependency.* New York: New Press.

Finnis, John (1980). *Natural Law and Natural Rights.* Oxford: Clarendon Press.

Fisher, Berenice and Joan Tronto (1990). 'Toward a Feminist Theory of Care', in Emily Abel and Margaret Nelson (eds), *Circles of Care: Work and Identity in Women's Lives.* Albany, NY: State University of New York Press, pp. 34–62.

Flanagan, Owen and J. Adler (1983). 'Impartiality and Particularity', *Social Research*, 50(3): 576–96.

Folbre, Nancy (1996). 'Roemer's Market Socialism: A Feminist Critique', in Erik Olin (ed.), *Equal Shares: Making Market Socialism Work.* London: Verso, pp. 57–70.

—— (2000). 'Universal Childcare: It's Time', *The Nation*, 271(1) (July 3).

—— (2001). *The Invisible Heart: Economics and Family Values.* New York: New Press.

—— (2006). "Demanding Quality: Worker/Consumer Coalitions and 'High Road' Strategies in the Care Sector," *Politics and Society*, 34(1): 11–32.

—— and Julie Nelson (2000). 'For Love or Money—Or Both?', *Journal of Economic Perspectives*, 14(4) (Fall): 123–40.

Fonagy, Peter (2001). *Attachment Theory and Psychoanalysis.* New York: Other Press.

Fowles, Jib (1999). *The Case for Television Violence.* Sage.

Franck, Thomas (2003). 'Interpretation and Change in the Law of Humanitarian Intervention', in J. L. Holzgrege and Robert Keohane (eds), *Humanitarian*

*Intervention: Ethical, Legal, and Political Dilemmas.* Cambridge: Cambridge University Press, pp. 204–31.

Fraser, Nancy and Axel Honneth (2003). *Redistribution or Recognition? A Political-Philosophical Exchange,* trans. Joel Golb, James Ingram, and Christiane Wilke. New York: Verso.

——— and Linda Gordon (2002). 'A Genealogy of Dependency: Tracing a Keyword of the U.S. Welfare State', in Eva Feder Kittay and Ellen Feder (eds), *The Subject of Care: Feminist Perspectives on Dependency.* Lanham, MD: Rowman and Littlefield, pp. 14–39.

Freedman, Jonathan (2002). *Media Violence and Its Effect on Aggression: Assessing the Scientific Evidence.* Toronto: University of Toronto Press.

Freeman, Michael (1994). 'The Philosophical Foundations of Human Rights', *Human Rights Quarterly,* 16: 491–514.

Friedman, Marilyn (1993). *What are Friends For? Feminist Perspectives on Personal Relationships and Moral Theory.* Ithaca, NY: Cornell University Press.

Friedman, Milton (1982). *Capitalism and Freedom.* Chicago, IL: University of Chicago Press.

Friedman, Richard (1981). 'The Basis of Human Rights: A Criticism of Gewirth's Theory', in J. Roland Pennock and John Chapman (eds), *NOMOS XXIII: Human Rights.* New York: New York University Press, pp. 148–57.

Friedman, Thomas (2000). *The Lexus and the Olive Tree.* New York: Anchor Books.

Galston, William (1995). 'A Liberal Case for the Two-Parent Family', in Amitai Etzioni (ed.), *Rights and the Common Good.* New York: St. Martin's Press.

Garbarino, James (1999). *Lost Boys: Why Our Sons Turn Violent and How We Can Save Them.* New York: Free Press.

——— and Aaron Ebata (1983). 'The Significance of Ethnic and Cultural Differences in Child Maltreatment', *Journal of Marriage and the Family,* 45(4) (November): 773–83.

Gardiner, Jean (1997). *Gender, Care and Economics.* London: Macmillan Press.

Gauthier, Anne (1996). *The State and the Family: A Comparative Analysis of Family Policies in Industrialized Countries.* Oxford: Clarendon Press.

Geen, Russell (2001). *Human Aggression,* 2nd edn, Philadelphia, PA: Open University Press.

Gerbner, George (1992). 'Violence and Terror in the Media', in Marc Raboy and Bernard Dagenais (eds), *Media, Crisis, and Democracy.* Newbury Park, CA: Sage, pp. 94–107.

——— (1995). 'Television Violence: The Power and the Peril', in Gail Dines and Jean Humez (eds), *Gender, Race, and Class in Media.* Thousand Oaks, CA: Sage, pp. 547–57.

Gewirth, Alan (1978). *Reason and Morality.* Chicago, IL: University of Chicago Press.

——— (1996). *The Community of Rights.* Chicago, IL: University of Chicago Press.

Gilens, Martin (1999). *Why Americans Hate Welfare: Race, Media, and the Politics of Antipoverty Policy.* Chicago, IL: University of Chicago Press.

Gilligan, Carol (1982). *In a Different Voice*. Cambridge, MA: Harvard University Press.

Gilligan, Carol (1986). 'Reply', *Signs*, 11(1) (Autumn): 324–33.

Goldberg, Susan (1977). 'Infant Development and Mother-Infant Interaction in Urban Zambia', in P. Herbert Liederman, Steven Tulkin, and Anne Rosenfeld (eds), *Culture and Infancy: Variations in the Human Experience*. New York: Academic Press, pp. 211–43.

Golding, Martin (1981). 'From Prudence to Rights: A Critique', in J. Roland Pennock and John Chapman (eds), *NOMOS XXIII: Human Rights*. New York: New York University Press, pp. 165–74.

Goleman, Daniel (1995). *Emotional Intelligence*. New York: Bantam Books.

Goodin, Robert (1985). *Protecting the Vulnerable: A Reanalysis of Our Social Responsibilities*. Chicago, IL: University of Chicago Press.

—— (1988). *Reasons for Welfare: The Political Theory of the Welfare State*. Princeton, NJ: Princeton University Press.

—— (1995). *Utilitarianism as a Public Philosophy*. Cambridge: Cambridge University Press.

—— (1996). 'Structures of Political Order: The Relational Feminist Alternative', *Political Order: NOMOS* 38: 498–521.

Gordon, Robert (2003). 'Exploding Productivity Growth: Context, Causes, and Implication', *Brookings Papers on Economic Activity*, 2: 207–98.

Gornick, Janet and Marcia Meyers (2003). *Families That Work: Policies for Reconciling Parenthood and Employment*. New York: Russell Sage Foundation.

Gould, Carol (2004). *Globalizing Democracy and Human Rights*. Cambridge: Cambridge University Press.

Gourevitch, Phillip (1998). *We Wish to Inform You that Tomorrow We Will be Killed with Our Families: Stories from Rwanda*. New York: Picador.

Greider, William (1997). *One World Ready or Not: The Manic Logic of Global Capitalism*. Simon and Schuster.

Grimshaw, Jean (1986). *Philosophy and Feminist Thinking*. Minneapolis, MN: University of Minnesota Press.

Groenhout, Ruth (2004). Connected Lives: Human Nature and an Ethics of Care. Lanham, MD: Rowman and Littlefield.

Grossman, Dave and Gloria Degaetano (1999). *Stop Teaching Our Kids to Kill: A Call to Action Against TV, Movie and Video Game Violence*. Crown: 1999.

Grossman, K. E., K. Grossman, and P. Zimmerman (1999). 'A Wider View of Attachment and Exploration', in J. Cassidy and P. R. Shaver (eds), *Handbook of Attachment: Theory, Research, and Clinical Applications*. New York: Guilford, pp. 760–86.

Habermas, Jurgen (1984). *The Theory of Communicative Action: Volume One: Reason and the Rationalization of Society*, trans. Thomas McCarthy. Boston, MA: Beacon Press.

____ (1987). *The Theory of Communicative Action: Volume Two: Lifeworld and System: A Critique of Functionalist Reason*. Trans. Thomas McCarthy. Boston, MA: Beacon Press.

____ (1990). *Moral Consciousness and Communicative Action*, trans. Christian Lenhardt and Shierry Weber Nicholsen. Cambridge, MA: MIT Press.

____ (1996). *Between Facts and Norms: Contributions to a Discourse Theory of Law and Democracy*, trans. William Rehg. Cambridge, MA: MIT Press.

Hahnel, Robin (1998). *Panic Rules! Everything You Need to Know about the Global Economy*. Cambridge, MA: South End Press.

Halwani, Raja (2003). 'Care Ethics and Virtue Ethics', *Hypatia*, 18(3) (Fall): 161–92.

Hamdi, Mohamed Elhachmi (1996). 'Islam and Liberal Democracy: The Limits of the Western Model', *Journal of Democracy*, 7(2): 81–5.

Hardesty, Constance, Deann Wenk, and Carolyn Stout Morgan (1995). 'Paternal Involvement and the Development of Gender Expectations in Sons and Daughters', *Youth and Society*, 26: 283–97.

Harrington, Mona (2000). *Care and Equality: Inventing a New Family Politics*. New York: Routledge.

Harris, Angela (1991). 'Race and Essentialism in Feminist Theory', in Katharine T. Bartlett and Roseanne Kennedy (eds), *Feminist Theory: Readings in Law and Gender*. Boulder, CO: Westview Press.

Haslett, D. W. (1994). *Capitalism and Morality*. Oxford: Clarendon Press.

Hays, Sharon (1996). *The Cultural Contradictions of Motherhood*. New Haven, CT: Yale University Press.

Headey, Bruce, Robert Goodin, Ruud Muffels, and Henk-Jan Dirven (2000). 'Is There a Trade-off between Economic Efficiency and a Generous Welfare State? A Comparison of Best Cases of "The Three Worlds of Welfare Capitalism"', *Social Indicators Research*, 50: 115–57.

Heath, Linda and Kevin Gilbert (1996). 'Mass Media and Fear of Crime', *American Behavioral Scientist*, 39(4) (February): 379–86.

Helburn, Suzanne and Barbara Bergmann (2002). *America's Child Care Problem: The Way Out*. New York: Palgrave.

Held, David (1995). *Democracy and the Global Order: From the Modern State to Cosmopolitan Governance*. Stanford, CA: Stanford University Press.

Held, Virginia (1984). *Rights and Goods: Justifying Social Action*. Chicago, IL: University of Chicago Press.

____ (1988). 'Access, Enablement, and the First Amendment', in Diana Meyers and Kenneth Kipnis (eds), *Philosophical Dimensions of the Constitution*. Boulder, CO: Westview Press.

____ (1993). *Feminist Morality: Transforming Culture, Society, and Politics*. Chicago, IL: University of Chicago Press.

____ (1995). 'The Meshing of Care and Justice', *Hypatia*, 10(2) (Spring): 128–32.

____ (2002). 'Care and the Extension of Markets', *Hypatia*, 17(2) (Spring): 19–33.

Held, Virginia (2006). *The Ethics of Care: Personal, Political, and Global.* Oxford: Oxford University Press.

Herrett-Skjellum, Jennifer and Mike Allen (1996). 'Television Programming and Sex Stereotyping: A Meta-Analysis', in Brant Burleson (ed.), *Communication Yearbook* 19. Thousand Oaks, CA: Sage, pp. 157–85.

Himmelweit, Susan (1999). 'Caring Labor', in Ronnie Steinberg and Deborah Figart (eds), *Emotional Labor in the Service Economy. The Annals of the American Academy of Political and Social Science* (January): 27–38.

Hirschmann, Nancy (1992). *Rethinking Obligation: A Feminist Method for Political Theory.* Ithaca, NY: Cornell University Press.

—— (1996). 'Revisioning Freedom: Relationship, Context, and the Politics of Empowerment', in Nancy Hirschmann and Christine Di Stefano (eds), *Revisioning the Political: Feminist Reconstructions of Traditional Concepts in Western Political Theory.* Boulder, CO: Westview Press, pp. 51–74.

—— (2003). *The Subject of Liberty: Toward a Feminist Theory of Freedom.* Princeton, NJ: Princeton University Press.

Hirst, Paul and Grahame Thompson (1999). *Globalization in Question,* 2nd edn, Cambridge: Polity Press.

Holmes, Stephen (1988). 'Liberal Guilt: Some Theoretical Origins of the Welfare State', in Donald Moon (ed.), *Responsibility, Rights, and Welfare: The Theory of the Welfare State.* Boulder, CO: Westview Press.

Holzgrefe, J. L. and Robert Keohane (eds) (2003). *Humanitarian Intervention: Ethical, Legal, and Political Dilemmas.* Cambridge: Cambridge University Press.

Hrdy, Sarah Blaffer (1999). *Mother Nature: A History of Mothers, Infants, and Natural Selection.* New York: Pantheon Books.

Huesmann, L. R. and L. S. Miller (1994). 'Long-term Effects of Repeated Exposure to Media Violence in Childhood', in L. R. Huesmann (ed.), *Aggressive Behavior: Current Perspectives.* New York: Plenum Press, pp. 153–86.

—— J. F. Moise, and C. Podolski (1997). 'The Effects of Media Violence on the Development of Antisocial Behavior', in D. Stoff, J. Breiling, and J. Maser (eds), *Handbook of Antisocial Behavior.* New York: Wiley, pp. 181–93.

—— J. Moise-Titus, C. L. Podolski, and L. D. Eron (2003). 'Longitudinal Relations between Children's Exposure to TV Violence and Their Aggressive and Violent Behavior in Young Adulthood: 1977–1992', *Developmental Psychology* 39(2): 201–21.

Hume, David (1983). *An Enquiry Concerning the Principles of Morals.* J. B. Schneewind (ed.). Indianapolis, IN: Hackett Publishing.

Huston, Aletha and John Wright (1998). 'Mass Media and Children's Development', in William Damon, Irving Siegel, and K. Anne Renninger, (eds) *Handbook of Child Psychology, Fifth Edition, Volume IV: Child Psychology in Practice.* New York: John Wiley and Sons, pp. 999–1058.

Iannotti, R. J., E M. Cummings, B. Pierrehumbert, M. J. Milano, and C. Zahn-Waxler (1992). 'Parental Influences on Prosocial Behavior and Empathy in Early

Childhood', in J. M. A. M. Janssens and J. R. M. Gerris (eds), *Child Rearing: Influence on Prosocial and Moral Development*. Amsterdam: Swets and Zeitlinger, pp. 77–100.

Ignatieff, Michael (2001). *Human Rights as Politics and Idolatry*. Princeton, NJ: Princeton University Press.

Isbister, John (2001). *Capitalism and Justice*. San Francisco, CA: Kumarian Press.

Iyengar, Shanto (1991). *Is Anyone Responsible? How Television Frames Political Issues*. Chicago, IL: University of Chicago Press.

Jaffee, Sara and Janet Shibley Hyde (2000). 'Gender Differences in Moral Orientation: A Meta-Analysis', *Psychological Bulletin*, 126(5): 703–26.

James, William (1991). *Pragmatism*. Amherst, NY: Prometheus Books.

Jochimsen, Maren (2003). *Careful Economics: Integrating Caring Activities and Economic Science*. Boston, MA: Kluwer Academic Publishers.

Johnson, D. W., R. T. Johnson and E. Holubec (1991). *Circles of Learning: Cooperation in the Classroom*. Edina, MN: Interaction Book Company.

Johnston, D. Kay (2006). *Education for a Caring Society: Classroom Relationships and Moral Action*. New York: Teachers College Press.

Jones, Charles (1999). *Global Justice: Defending Cosmopolitanism*. Oxford: Oxford University Press.

Kausikan, Bilahari (1993). 'Asia's Different Standard', *Foreign Policy*, 92: 24–41.

Kennedy, David (2004). *The Dark Side of Virtue: Reassessing International Humanitarianism*. Princeton, NJ: Princeton University Press.

Keohane, Robert (2003). 'Political Authority after Intervention: Gradations in Sovereignty', in Holzgrefe, J. L. and Robert Keohane (eds), *Humanitarian Intervention: Ethical, Legal, and Political Dilemmas*. Cambridge: Cambridge University Press, pp. 275–98.

Kestenbaum, R., E. A. Faber, and L. A. Sroufe (1989). 'Individual Differences in Empathy among Preschoolers: Relation to Attachment History', in Nancy Eisenberg (ed.), *New Directions for Child Development, Volume 44: Empathy and Related Emotional Responses*. San Francisco, CA: Jossey-Bass, pp. 51–64.

Kirp, David (2004). 'Life Way After Head Start', *New York Times Magazine*, 21 (November): 32–8.

Kittay, Eva Feder (1999). *Love's Labor: Essays on Women, Equality, and Dependency*. New York: Routledge.

—— (2001). 'A Feminist Public Ethic of Care Meets the New Communitarian Family Policy', *Ethics*, 111 (April): 523–47.

—— and Ellen K. Feder (eds) (2002). *The Subject of Care: Feminist Perspectives on Dependency*. Lanham, MD: Rowman and Littlefield.

—— Bruce Jennings, and Angela Wasunna (2005). 'Dependency, Difference, and the Global Ethic of Longterm Care', *The Journal of Political Philosophy*, 13(4): 443–69.

Klosko, George (1992). *The Principle of Fairness and Political Obligation*. Lanham, MD: Rowman and Littlefield.

Koester, R., C. Franz, and J. Weinberger (1990). 'The Family Origins of Empathic Concern: A 26-Year Longitudinal Study', *Journal of Personality and Social Psychology*, 58: 709–17.

Konner, Melvin (1977). 'Infancy among the Kalahari Desert San', in P. Herbert Liederman, Steven Tulkin, and Anne Rosenfeld (eds), *Culture and Infancy: Variations in the Human Experience*. New York: Academic Press, pp. 287–328.

Korbin, Jill (1977). 'Anthropological Contributions to the Study of Child Abuse', *Child Abuse and Neglect*, 1: 7–24.

—— (1979). 'A Cross-Cultural Perspective on the Role of the Community in Child Abuse and Neglect', *Child Abuse and Neglect*, 3: 9–18.

—— (ed.) (1981). *Child Abuse and Neglect: Cross-Cultural Perspectives*. Berkeley, CA: University of California Press.

—— (1982). 'What is Acceptable and Unacceptable Child-Rearing—A Cross-Cultural Consideration', in Kim Oates (ed.), *Child Abuse: A Community Concern*. New York: Brunner/Mazel.

Koren, Charlotte (2004). 'Who Cares?', *Feminist Economics*, 10(2): 258–61.

Kremer, Michael and Seema Jayachandran (2006). 'Odious Debt', *American Economic Review*, 96(1) (March): 82–92.

Kurtz, Stanley (1992). *All the Mothers are One: Hindu India and the Cultural Reshaping of Psychoanalysis*. New York: Columbia University Press.

Kusche, Carol, and Mark Greenberg (2001). 'PATHS in Your Classroom: Promoting Emotional Literacy and Alleviating Emotional Distress', in Jonathan Cohen (ed.), *Caring Classrooms/Intelligent Schools: The Social Emotional Education of Young Children*. New York: Teachers College Press, pp. 140–61.

Kuttner, Robert (1997). *Everything for Sale: The Virtues and Limits of Markets*. New York: Alfred Knopf.

Kymlicka, Will (1990). *Contemporary Political Philosophy: An Introduction*. Oxford: Clarendon Press.

—— (1995). *Multicultural Citizenship: A Liberal Theory of Minority Rights*. Oxford: Clarendon Press.

Lamb, Michael (1998). 'Nonparental Child Care: Context, Quality, Correlations, and Consequences', in William Damon, Irving Siegel, and K. Anne Renninger (eds), *Handbook of Child Psychology, Fifth Edition, Volume 4: Child Psychology in Practice*. New York: John Wiley and Sons, pp. 73–133.

Lappe, Frances Moore and Joseph Collins (1986). *World Hunger: Twelve Myths*. New York: Grove Press.

Lauren, Paul Gordon (1998). *The Evolution of International Human Rights: Visions Seen*. Philadelphia, PA: University of Pennsylvania Press.

Levinas, Emmanuel (1969). *Totality and Infinity: An Essay on Exteriority*. Trans. Alphonso Lingis. Pittsburgh, PA: Duquesne University Press.

Levine, Robert (1977). 'Child Rearing as Cultural Adaptation', in P. Herbert Liederman, Steven Tulkin, and Anne Rosenfeld (eds), *Culture and Infancy: Variations in the Human Experience*. New York: Academic Press.

Lewis, Michael and Peggy Ban (1977). 'Variance and Invariance in the Mother-Infant Interaction: A Cross-Cultural Study', in P. Herbert Liederman, Steven Tulkin, and Anne Rosenfeld (eds), *Culture and Infancy: Variations in the Human Experience*. New York: Academic Press, pp. 329–55.

Liederman, P. Herbert, Steven Tulkin, and Anne Rosenfeld (eds) (1977). *Culture and Infancy: Variations in the Human Experience*. New York: Academic Press.

Linz, D. G., E. Donnerstein, and S. Penrod (1988). 'Effects of Long-term Exposure to Violent and Sexually Degrading Depictions of Women', *Journal of Personality and Social Psychology*, 55: 758–68.

Luke, Brian (1996). 'Justice, Caring, and Animal Liberation', in Josephine Donovan and Carol Adams (eds), *Beyond Animal Rights: A Feminist Ethic for the Treatment of Animals*. New York: Continuum, pp. 77–102.

Lyons-Ruth, K (1996). 'Attachment Relationships among Children with Aggressive Behavior Problems: The Role of Disorganized Early Attachment Patterns', *Journal of Consulting and Clinical Psychology*, 64: 32–40.

Maccoby, Eleanor and Catherine Lewis (2003). 'Less Day Care or Different Day Care?', *Child Development*, 74(4) 1069–75.

MacIntyre, Alasdair (1981). *After Virtue*. Notre Dame, IN: University of Notre Dame Press.

—— (1999). *Dependent Rational Animals: Why Human Beings Need the Virtues*. Chicago, IL: Open Court.

Malamuth, N. M. and J. V. P. Check (1981). 'The Effects of Mass Media Exposure on Acceptance of Violence against Women: A Field Experiment', *Journal of Research in Personality*, 15: 436–46.

Mapel, David and Terry Nardin (eds) (1998). *International Society: Diverse Ethical Perspectives*. Princeton, NJ: Princeton University Press.

Maren, Michael (1997). *The Road to Hell: The Ravaging Effects of Foreign Aid and International Charity*. New York: Free Press.

Marx, Karl (1976). *Capital, volume I*. London: Lawrence and Wishart.

Masse, L. and W. S. Barnett (2002). 'A Benefit Cost Analysis of the Abecedarian Early Childhood Intervention'. New Jersey: National Institute for Early Education Research. Available athttp://nieer.org/resources/research/AbecedarianStudy.pdf#search =%22masse%20and%20barnett%22

Mayer, Ann Elizabeth (1991). *Islam and Human Rights*. Boulder, CO: Westview Press.

McLaren, Margaret (2001). 'Feminist ethics: Care as Virtue', in Peggy DesAutels and Joanne Waugh (eds), *Feminists Doing Ethics*. Lanham, MD: Rowman and Littlefield.

Meagher, Gabrielle and Julie Nelson (2004). 'Survey Article: Feminism in the Dismal Science', *The Journal of Political Philosophy*, 12(1): 102–26.

Meyers, Diana (1993). 'Moral Reflection: Beyond Impartial Reason', *Hypatia*, 8(3) (Summer): 21–47.

Midgley, Mary (1984). *Animals and Why They Matter*. Athens, GA: University of Georgia Press.

257

Mies, Maria and Vandana Shiva (1993). *Ecofeminism*. London: Zed Books.

Miller, David (1989). *Market, State, and Community*. Oxford: Clarendon Press.

Miller, Matthew (2003). *The Two Percent Solution: Fixing America's Problems in Ways Liberals and Conservatives Can Love*. New York: Public Affairs.

Minow, Martha (1990). *Making All the Difference: Inclusion, Exclusion, and American Law*. Ithaca, NY: Cornell University Press.

Monroe, Kristin Renwick (2004). *The Hand of Compassion: Portraits of Moral Choice During the Holocaust*. Princeton, NJ: Princeton University Press.

Moon, J. Donald (1988). 'The Moral Basis of the Democratic Welfare State', in Amy Gutman (ed.), *Democracy and the Welfare State*. Princeton, NJ: Princeton University Press.

Morgan, M. and J. Shanahan (1997). 'Two Decades of Cultivation Research', in B. R. Burleson and A. W. Kunkel (eds), *Communication Yearbook 20*. Thousand Oaks, CA: Sage, pp. 1–45.

Morris, Arval (1981). 'A Differential Theory of Human Rights', in J. Roland Pennock and John Chapman (eds), *NOMOS XXIII: Human Rights*. New York: New York University Press, pp. 158–64.

Murray, Charles (1984). *Losing Ground: American Social Policy, 1950–1980*. New York: Basic Books.

Mussen, Paul and Nancy Eisenberg-Berg (1977). *Roots of Caring, Sharing, and Helping: The Development of Prosocial Behavior in Children*. San Francisco, CA: W. H. Freeman and Company.

Narayan, Uma (1995). 'Colonialism and Its Others: Considerations on Rights and Care Discourses', *Hypatia*, 10(2): 133–40.

Nardin, Terry and David Mapel (1992). *Traditions of International Ethics*. Cambridge: Cambridge University Press.

National Education Association (2003). *Status of the American Public School Teacher 2000–2001*. Washington, DC: National Educational Association. Available at http://www.nea.org/edstats/images/status.pdf

Nelson, Julie (1993). 'The Study of Choice or the Study of Provisioning? Gender and the Definition of Economics', in M. A. Ferber and J. Nelson (eds), *Beyond Economic Man: Feminist Theory and Economics*. Chicago, IL: University of Chicago Press, pp. 23–36.

—— (2006). 'Can We Talk? Feminist Economists in Dialogue with Social Theorists', *Signs: Journal of Women in Culture and Society*, 31(4) (Summer): 1051–74.

Noddings, Nel (1984). *Caring: A Feminine Approach to Ethics and Moral Education*. Berkeley, CA: University of California Press.

—— (1992). *The Challenge to Care in Schools: An Alternative Approach to Education*. New York: Teachers College Press.

—— (2002). *Starting at Home: Caring and Social Policy*. Berkeley, CA: University of California Press.

—— (2003). *Happiness and Education*. Cambridge: Cambridge University Press.

Nozick, Robert (1974). *Anarchy, State, and Utopia*. New York: Basic Books.

Nussbaum, Martha (2000). *Women and Human Development: The Capabilities Approach*. Cambridge: Cambridge University Press.

_____ (2001). *Upheavals of Thought: The Intelligence of the Emotions*. Cambridge: Cambridge University Press.

O'Brien, Ruth (2005). *Bodies in Revolt: Gender, Disability, and a Workplace Ethic of Care*. New York: Routledge.

Offe, Claus (1988). 'Democracy Against the Welfare State? Structural Foundations of Neoconservative Political Opportunities', in J. Donald Moon (ed.), *Responsibility, Rights, and Welfare: The Theory of the Welfare State*. Boulder, CO: Westview Press, pp. 189–228.

Okin, Susan (1989*a*). *Justice, Gender, and the Family*. New York: Basic Books.

_____ (1989*b*). 'Reason and Feeling in Thinking about Justice', *Ethics*, 99: 229–49.

_____ (1990). 'Thinking Like a Woman', in Deborah Rhode (ed.), *Theoretical Perspectives on Sexual Difference*. New Haven, CT: Yale University Press.

_____ (2003). 'Poverty, Well-Being, and Gender: What Counts, Who's Heard?', *Philosophy and Public Affairs*, 31(3) (Summer): 280–316.

Oliner, Pearl (1979). 'Compassion and Caring: Missing Concepts in Social Studies Programs', *Journal of Education*, 161 (Fall): 36–60.

_____ (1983). 'Putting "Community" into Citizenship Education: The Need for Prosociality', *Theory and Research in Social Education*, 11(2): 65–81.

_____ (1985/6). 'Legitimating and Implementing Prosocial Education', *Humboldt Journal of Social Relations*, 13(1 & 2): 391–410.

Oliner, Samuel and Pearl Oliner (1988). *The Altruistic Personality: Rescuers of Jews in Nazi Europe*. New York: Free Press.

Ollman, Bertell (1979). *Social and Sexual Revolution*. Boston, MA: South End Press.

_____ (ed.) (1998). *Market Socialism: The Debate Among Socialists*. New York: Routledge.

Olson, Emelie (1981). 'Socioeconomic and Psycho-Cultural Contexts of Child Abuse and Neglect in Turkey', in Korbin, Jill (ed.), *Child Abuse and Neglect: Cross-Cultural Perspectives*. Berkeley, CA: University of California Press, pp. 96–119.

O'Neill, Onora (1992). 'Justice, Gender, and International Boundaries,' in Robin Attfield and Barry Wilkins (eds), *International Justice and the Third World*. New York: Routledge, pp. 50–76.

Pally, Marcia (1994). *Sex and Sensibility: Reflections on Forbidden Mirrors and the Will to Censor*. New Jersey: ECCO Press.

Parekh, Bhikhu (2000). *Rethinking Multiculturalism: Cultural Diversity and Political Theory*. Cambridge, MA: Harvard University Press.

Physicians' Working Group for Single-Payer National Health Insurance (2003). 'Proposal of the Physicians' Working Group for Single-Payer National Health Insurance', *JAMA: The Journal of the American Medical Association*, 290(6) (August 13): 798–805.

Pogge, Thomas (2002). *World Poverty and Human Rights*. Cambridge: Polity Press.

Polanyi, Karl (2001). *The Great Transformation: The Political and Economic Origins of Our Time*. Boston, MA: Beacon Press.

Pollack, William (1998). *Real Boys*. New York: Henry Holt and Company.

Pollis, Adamantia (1996). 'Cultural Relativism Revisited: Through a State Prism', *Human Rights Quarterly*, 18: 316–44.

—— and Peter Schwab (1979). 'Human Rights: A Western Construct with Limited Applicability', in Adamantia Pollis and Peter Schwab (eds), *Human Rights: Cultural and Ideological Perspectives*. New York: Praeger, pp. 1–18.

Popenoe, David (1996). *Life Without Father*. New York: Free Press.

Potter, W. James (2003). *The 11 Myths of Media Violence*. Thousand Oaks, CA: Sage.

Puka, Bill (1990). 'The Liberation of Caring: A Different Voice For Gilligan's "Different Voice" ', *Hypatia*, 55(1): 58–82.

—— (1991). 'Interpretative Experiments: Probing the Care-Justice Debate in Moral Development', *Human Development*, (34): 61–80.

Putnam, Robert (2000). *Bowling Alone: The Collapse and Revival of American Community*. New York: Simon and Schuster.

Radke-Yarrow, M. and C. Zahn-Waxler (1986). 'The Role of Familial Factors in the Development of Prosocial Behavior: Research Findings and Questions', in Dan Olweus, Jack Block, and Marian Radke-Yarrow (eds), *Development of Antisocial and Prosocial Behavior: Research, Theories, and Issues*. Orlando, FL: Academic Press, pp. 207–33.

Rank, Mark (2004). *One Nation, Underprivileged: Why American Poverty Affects Us All*. Oxford: Oxford University Press.

Rawls, John (1996). *Political Liberalism*. New York: Columbia University Press.

—— (1999a). *The Law of Peoples*. Cambridge, MA: Harvard University Press.

—— (1999b). *A Theory of Justice*. Cambridge, MA: Harvard University Press.

Reader, Soran (2006). 'Does a Basic Needs Approach Need Capabilities?', *The Journal of Political Philosophy*, 14 (3): 337–50.

Regan, Tom (1991). *Thee Generation: Reflections on the Coming Revolution*. Philadelphia, PA: Temple University Press.

Reich, Robert (1992). *The Work of Nations*. New York: Vintage Books.

Renteln, Alison Dundes (1990). *International Human Rights: Universalism versus Relativism*. Newbury Park, CA: Sage Publications.

—— (2004). *The Cultural Defense*. Oxford: Oxford University Press.

The Responsive Communitarian Platform: Rights and Responsibilities (1998). In Amitai Etzioni (ed.), *The Essential Communitarian Reader*. Lanham, MD: Rowman and Littlefield.

Reynolds, Arthur, Judy Temple, Dylan Robertson, and Emily Mann (2001). 'Age 21 Cost–Benefit Analysis of the Title 1 Chicago Child-Parent Center Program'. At http://www.waisman.wisc.edu/cls/Chicago.htm

Rishmawi, Mona (1996). 'The Arab Charter on Human Rights: A Comment', *Interights Bulletin*, 10(1): 8–10.

Roberts, Dorothy (2002). 'Poverty, Race, and the Distortion of Dependency: The Case of Kinship Care', in Eva Feder Kittay and Ellen Feder (eds), *The Subject of Care*. Lanham, MD: Rowman and Littlefield, pp. 277–93.

Robinson, Fiona (1999). *Globalizing Care: Ethics, Feminist Theory, and International Relations*. Boulder, CO: Westview.

Roemer, John (1996). *Equal Shares: Making Market Socialism Work*. New York: Verso.

Rorty, Richard (1989). *Contingency, Irony, and Solidarity*. Cambridge: Cambridge University Press.

Rothstein, Bo (1998). *Just Institutions Matter: The Moral and Political Logic of the Universal Welfare State*. Cambridge: Cambridge University Press.

____ (2005). *Social Traps and the Problem of Trust*. Cambridge: Cambridge University Press.

____ Eric Uslaner (2005). 'All for All: Equality, Corruption, and Social Trust', *World Politics*, 58 (October): 41–72.

Ruddick, Sara (1989). *Maternal Politics: Toward a Politics of Peace*. Boston, MA: Beacon.

Sambasivan, Umadevi (2001). 'Development, Freedom, and Care: The Case of India', in Mary Daly (ed.), *Care Work: The Quest for Security*. Geneva: International Labour Office, pp. 79–90.

Sandel, Michael (1982). *Liberalism and the Limits of Justice*. Cambridge: Cambridge University Press.

Scanlon, T. M (1998). *What We Owe to Each Other*. Cambridge, MA: Harvard University Press.

Scarr, Sandra and Marlene Eisenberg (1993). 'Child Care Reasearch: Issues, Perspectives, and Results', *Annual Review of Psychology*, 44: 613–44.

Scheper-Hughes, Nancy (1992). *Death Without Weeping: The Violence of Everyday Life in Brazil*. Berkeley, CA: University of California Press.

Schwarzenbach, Sibyl (1987). 'Rawls and Ownership: The Forgotten Category of Reproductive Labor', in Marsha Hanen and Kai Nielsen (eds), *Science, Morality, and Feminist Theory. Supplementary Volume of the Canadian Journal of Philosophy*. Calgary, Canada: University of Calgary Press.

____ (1996). 'On Civic Friendship', *Ethics*, 107 (October): 97–128.

Schweickart, David (1993). *Against Capitalism*. Cambridge: Cambridge University Press.

____ (1998). 'Market Socialism: A Defense', in Bertell Ollman (ed.), *Market Socialism: The Debate Among Socialists*. New York: Routledge.

____ (2002). *After Capitalism*. Lanham, MD: Rowman and Littlefield.

Schweinhart, L. J. (2004). *The High/Scope Perry Preschool Study Through Age 40: Summary, Conclusions, and Frequently Asked Questions*. Ypsilanti, MI: High/Scope Press.

____ J. Montie, Z. Xiang, W. S. Barnett, C.R. Belfield, and M. Nores (2005). *Lifetime Effects: The High/Scope Perry Preschool Study Through Age 40*. Ypsilanti, MI: High/Scope Press. The study is available at www.highscope.org/welcome.asp

Seccombe, Wally (1974). 'The Housewife and Her Labour under Capitalism', *New Left Review*, 83 (January–February): 3–24.

Sen, Amartya (1984). *Resources, Values, and Development*. Cambridge, MA: Harvard University Press.

—— (1987). *The Standard of Living*. Edited by Geoffrey Hawthorn. Cambridge: Cambridge University Press.

—— (1999). *Development as Freedom*. New York: Random House.

Sevenhuijsen, Selma (1998). *Citizenship and the Ethics of Care*. Trans. Liz Savage. New York: Routledge.

Shachar, Ayelet (2001). *Multicultural Jurisdictions: Cultural Differences and Women's Rights*. Cambridge: Cambridge University Press.

Shaw, D. S., E. B. Owens, J. I. Vondra, K. Keenan, and W. B. Winslow (1997). 'Early Risk Factors and Pathways in the Development of Early Disruptive Behavior Problems', *Developmental and Psychopathology*, 8: 679–99.

—— and J. I. Vondra (1995). 'Infant Attachment Security and Maternal Predictors of Early Behavior Problems: A Longitudinal Study of Low-Income Families', *Journal of Abnormal Child Psychology*, 23: 335–57.

Shields, Vickie Rutledge (1997). 'Selling the Sex that Sells: Mapping the Evolution of Gender Advertising Research Across Three Decades', in Brant Burleson (ed.), *Communication Yearbook 20*. Thousand Oaks, CA: Sage, pp. 71–109.

Shue, Henry (1996). *Basic Rights: Subsistence, Affluence, and U.S. Foreign Policy*, 2nd edn, Princeton, NJ: Princeton University Press.

Shure, Myrna and Ann-Linn Glaser (2001). 'I Can Problem Solve (ICPS): A Cognitive Approach to the Prevention of Early High-Risk Behaviors', in Jonathan Cohen (ed.), *Caring Classrooms/Intelligent Schools: The Social Emotional Education of Young Children*. New York: Teachers College Press, pp. 122–39.

Siegel, Daniel (1999). *The Developing Mind: Toward a Neurobiology of Interpersonal Experience*. New York: Guilford Press.

Signorielli, Nancy (1990). 'Television's Mean and Dangerous World', in Nancy Signorielli and Michael Morgan, (eds), *Cultivation Analysis*. Newbury Park, CA: Sage, pp. 85–106.

Silk, John (1998). 'Caring at a Distance', *Ethics, Peace, and Environment*, 1(2): 165–82.

Simmons, A. John (1979). *Moral Principles and Political Obligations*. Princeton, NJ: Princeton University Press.

Singer, Peter (1993). *Practical Ethics*. Cambridge: Cambridge University Press.

—— (2002). *One World: The Ethics of Globalization*. New Haven, CT: Yale University Press.

Slavin, R. E (1990). *Cooperative Learning: Theory, Research, and Practice*. Englewood Cliffs, NJ: Prentice Hall.

Smith, Paul (1978). 'Domestic Labour and Marx's Theory of Value', in Annette Kuhn and AnnMarie Wolpe (eds), *Feminism and Materialism: Women and Modes of Production*. London: Routledge and Kegan Paul.

Slote, Michael (2001). *Morals from Motives*. Oxford: Oxford University Press.

Solomon, Robert (1995). *A Passion for Justice: Emotions and the Origins of the Social Contract*. Lanham, MD: Rowman and Littlefield.

Sroufe, L. A. (1983). 'Infant-Caregiver Attachment and Patterns of Adaptation in Preschool: The Roots of Maladaptation and Competence', in M. Perlmutter (ed.), *Development and Policy Concerning Children with Special Needs. Minnesota Symposia on Child Psychology. Volume 16*. Hillsdale, NJ: Erlbaum, pp. 41–83.

Staub, E (1992). 'The Origins of Caring, Helping and Nonaggression: Parental Socialization, the Family System, Schools and Cultural Influence', in S. Oliner, P. Oliner, L. Baron, L. A. Blu, D. L. Krebs, and M. Z. Smolenaska (eds), *Embracing the Other: Philosophical, Pscyhological and Historical Perspectives on Altruism*. New York: New York University Press, pp. 390–412.

Steger, Manfred (2002). *Globalism: The New Market Ideology*. Lanham, MD: Rowman and Littlefield.

Streeten, Paul, with Shahid Javed Burki, Mahbub Ul Haq, Norman Hicks, and Frances Stewart (1981). *First Things First: Meeting Basic Human Needs in Developing Countries*. Oxford: Oxford University Press.

Streuning, Karen (2002). *New Family Values: Liberty, Equality, Diversity*. Lanham, MD: Rowman and Littlefield.

Stewart, Frances (2006). 'The Basic Needs Approach', in D. A. Clark (ed.), *The Elgar Companion to Development Studies*. Cheltenham, UK: Edward Elgar.

Stiglitz, Joseph (2002). *Globalization and Its Discontents*. New York: W. W. Norton and Company.

Tamm, Ingrid (2004). 'Dangerous Appetites: Human Rights Activism and Conflict Commodities', *Human Rights Quarterly*, 26: 687–704.

Tan, Kok-Chor (2000). *Toleration, Diversity, and Global Justice*. University Park, PA: Pennsylvania State University Press.

Tang, James T. H. (ed.) (1995). *Human Rights and International Relations in the Asia Pacific*. London: Pinter.

Taylor, Charles (1994). *Multiculturalism: Examining the Politics of Recognition*. Princeton, NJ: Princeton University Press.

—— (1985). *Philosophy and the Human Sciences: Philosophical Papers 2*. Cambridge: Cambridge University Press.

Thomas, Aquinas, Saint (2002). *On Law, Morality, and Politics*, 2nd edn, trans. Richard Regan. Indianapolis, IN: Hackett Publishing.

Thompson, Ross (1998). 'Early Sociopersonality Development', in William Damon and Nancy Eisenberg (eds), *Handbook of Child Psychology. Volume Three: Social, Emotional, and Personality Development*. New York: John Wiley and Sons, pp. 25–104.

Tibi, Bassam (1994). 'Islamic Law/Shari'a, Human Rights, Universal Morality and International Relations', *Human Rights Quarterly*, 16: 277–99.

Tronto, Joan (1987). 'Beyond Gender Difference to a Theory of Care', *Signs: Journal of Women in Culture and Society*, 12(4): 644–63.

Tronto, Joan (1993). *Moral Boundaries: A Political Argument for an Ethic of Care.* New York: Routledge.

—— (1996). 'Care as a Political Concept', in Nancy Hirschmann and Christine Di Stefano (eds), *Revisioning the Political: Feminist Reconstructions of Traditional Concepts in Western Political Theory.* Boulder, CO: Westview Press, pp. 139–56.

—— (1998). 'An Ethic of Care', *Generations*, 22(3) (Fall): 15–21.

U.S. Census Bureau (2005). *Statistical Abstract of the United States: 2006,* 125th edn, Washington, DC: U.S. Government Printing Office. Available at http://www.census.gov/compendia/statab/labor_force_employment_earnings/labor.pdf

Uslaner, Eric (1998). 'Social Capital, Television, and the "Mean World": Trust, Optimism, and Civic Participation', *Political Psychology*, 19(3) (September): 441–67.

—— (2002). *The Moral Foundations of Trust.* Cambridge: Cambridge University Press.

Valadez, Jorge (2001). *Deliberative Democracy, Political Legitimacy, and Self-Determination in Multicultural Societies.* Boulder, CO: Westview.

Van Lange, Paul A., Ellen M. N. De Bruin, Wilma Otten, and Jeffrey A. Joireman (1997). 'Development of Prosocial, Individualistic, and Competitive Orientations: Theory and Preliminary Evidence', *Journal of Personality and Social Psychology*, 73(4): 733–46.

Van Parijs, Philippe (1998). *Real Freedom for All: What (if anything) Can Justify Capitalism?* Clarendon: Oxford.

Vincent, R. J (1986). *Human Rights and International Relations.* Cambridge: Cambridge University Press.

Waerness, Kari (1984). 'Caring as Women's Work in the Welfare State', in Harriet Holter (ed.), *Patriarchy in a Welfare Society.* Oslo: Universitetsforlaget.

—— (1987). 'On the Rationality of Caring', in Anne Showstack Sassoon (ed.), *Women and the State: The Shifting Boundaries of Public and Private.* London: Hutchinson.

Walker, Margaret Urban (1998). *Moral Understandings.* New York: Routledge.

Waring, Marilyn (1988). *If Women Counted: A New Feminist Economics.* New York: HarperCollins.

Warren, Karen (2000). *Ecofeminist Philosophy: A Western Perspective on What It Is and Why It Matters.* Lanham, MD: Rowman and Littlefield.

Waters, E., D. Hay, and J. Richters (1986). 'Infant-Parent Attachment and the Origins of Prosocial and Antisocial Behavior', in Dan Olweus, Jack Block, and Marian Radke-Yarrow (eds), *Development of Antisocial and Prosocial Behavior: Research, Theories, and Issues.* Orlando, FL: Academic Press, pp. 97–125.

—— J. Wippmann, and L. A. Sroufe (1979). 'Attachment, Positive Affect, and Competence in the Peer Group: Two Studies in Construct Validation', *Child Development*, 50: 821–9.

Weinfield, N. S., L. A. Sroufe, B. Egeland, and A. E. Carlson (1999). 'The Nature of Individual Differences in Infant-Caregiver Attachment', in J. Cassidy and P. R.

Shaver (eds), *Handbook of Attachment: Theory, Research and Clinical Applications*. New York: Guilford, pp. 68–88.

Weiss, Thomas (1998). 'Principles, Politics, and Humanitarian Action', *Humanitarianism and War Project*. URL: http://hwproject.tufts.edu/publications/ electronic/e_ppaha.html

Wenar, Leif (2003). 'What We Owe to Distant Others', *Politics, Philosophy, and Economics*, 2(3): 283–304.

West, Robin (1997). *Caring for Justice*. New York: New York University Press.

____ (2002). 'The Right to Care', in Eva Feder Kittay and Ellen Feder (eds), *The Subject of Care: Feminist Perspectives on Dependency*. Lanham, MD: Rowman and Littlefield.

White, Julie Ann (2000). *Democracy, Justice, and the Welfare State*. University Park, Pennsylvania: PA State University Press.

____ and Joan Tronto (2004). 'Political Practices of Care: Needs and Rights', *Ratio Juris*, 17(4) (December): 425–53.

Whitehead, Barbara Defoe (1993). 'Dan Quayle Was Right', *The Atlantic*, 271(4): 47–84.

Whitman, Walt (1980). *Leaves of Grass: A Textual Variorum of the Printed Poems*. Volume I. New York: New York University Press.

Wiggins, David (1998). *Needs, Values, Truth: Essays in the Philosophy of Value*. Oxford: Clarendon Press.

Williams, Edith, Norma Radin, and Theresa Allegro (1992). 'Sex Role Attitudes of Adolescents Reared Primarily by Their Fathers: An 11-Year Follow-Up', *Merrill-Palmer Quarterly*, 38: 457–76.

Williams, Joan (2000). *Unbending Gender*. Oxford: Oxford University Press.

Winnicott, Donald (1965). *The Maturational Process and the Facilitating Environment: Studies in the Theory of Emotional Development*. London: Hogarth Press and the Institute of Psychoanalysis.

Young, Iris Marion (1990). *Justice and the Politics of Difference*. Princeton, NJ: Princeton. University Press.

____ (2002). 'Autonomy, Welfare Reform, and Meaningful Work', in Eva Feder Kittay and Ellen Feder (eds), *The Subject of Care: Feminist Perspectives on Dependency*. Lanham, MD: Rowman and Littlefield, pp. 40–60.

Zakaria, Fareed (1994). 'Culture is Destiny: A Conversation with Lee Kuan Yew', *Foreign Affairs*, 73(2): 109–26.

Zillmann, D. and J. Bryant (1982). 'Pornography, Sexual Callousness, and the Trivialization of Rape', *Journal of Communication*, 32(4): 10–21.

# Index

CPSIA information can be obtained at www.ICGtesting.com
Printed in the USA
LVOW070733260812

295956LV00002B/20/P